PHARMACIST'S GUIDE

— TO —

OVER-THE-COUNTER

— AND —

NATURAL REMEDIES

ROBERT GARRISON, JR., RPh

MICHAEL MANNION

AVERY PUBLISHING GROUP

Garden City Park • New York

The information and procedures contained in this book are based upon the research and the personal and professional experiences of the authors. They are not intended as a substitute for consulting with your physician or other health-care providers. The publisher and the authors are not responsible for any adverse effects or consequences resulting from the use of any of the suggestions, preparations, or treatment therapies discussed in this book. All matters pertaining to your physical health should be supervised by a health-care professional.

ISBN 0–89529–850–3

Printed in the United States of America

10 9 8 7 6 5 4 3 2 1

Contents

PART ONE: Learning About Over-the-Counter and Natural Remedies

PART TWO: An A-to-Z Guide to Common Conditions

APPENDICES

*To Tami Coyne, a hard-working editor,
a wonderful writer, and a great friend.*

— MM

Acknowledgments

We wish to express our gratitude and appreciation to our editor at Avery, Helene Ciaravino, for the creativity and hard work she brought to our project. Helene's editorial work was invaluable and helped make our book even more useful to our readers.

Preface

The Pharmacist's Guide to Over-the-Counter and Natural Remedies is your guide to two worlds of medical self-care. This book is a bridge that will help you make informed choices between the familiar drugstore medications and the available herbs, vitamins, minerals, and other natural substances that can be used for medicinal purposes. Importantly, these two worlds are not competitors. Our goal is not to promote one type of treatment over another, but to inform you about your options, and about the benefits and side effects that each option involves. We aim to help you make the best decision about how to manage your specific condition.

Part One of this book addresses the basics on managing conditions that don't require a doctor's close monitoring. It offers definitions, guidelines, and precautions concerning self-treatment of symptoms; tips on properly using and storing your remedies; pointers on how to choose a pharmacist; advice on the managing of children's illnesses; and much more. We include material on daily vitamin/mineral supplementation, and even helpful information on possible interactions between herbs and drugs.

Part Two discusses over seventy-five conditions, defining the conditions themselves and making valuable suggestions for treatment. Both OTC (over-the-counter) and natural remedies are recommended, and necessary precautions are addressed. All information is categorized under the alphabetical listing of conditions. (There is also an index at the back of the book, which will be helpful in case you are searching for a condition under another common name.) Easy-to-use charts put dosages and warnings at your fingertips. Of course, if you find that your symptoms are worsening, or are simply not improving, you should contact a physician for guidance. Furthermore, any questions or reservations that you may have are legitimate and should be discussed with a health-care professional.

This book offers you the most authoritative, up-to-date information on how to use the wide range of drug-store OTC and natural remedies. You don't have to rely on commercials and ads that give you only half the story. You don't have to go blindly and hesitantly into the natural products aisle. *The Pharmacist's Guide to Over-the-Counter and Natural Remedies* is a helpful handbook and a thorough reference tool that can help you take the surest steps in finding relief for yourself and your loved ones.

Codes and
Abbreviations

g	gram(s)
IU	international unit(s)
MCU	milkclotting unit(s)
mcg	microgram(s)
mg	milligram(s)
oz	ounce(s)
tbsp	tablespoon(s)
tsp	teaspoon(s)
+	plus; and greater
>	greater than
<	less than

PART ONE

Learning About Over-the-Counter and Natural Remedies

When it comes to selecting, purchasing, using, and storing over-the-counter (OTC) and natural remedies, there's a lot to learn. What should I look for on an OTC label? What forms do natural remedies come in? Should I store my medicines in my bathroom medicine cabinet? What precautions are necessary when giving children remedies?

Don't be overwhelmed. Part One of *The Pharmacist's Guide to Over-the-Counter and Natural Remedies* gives you fast and easy answers. Each section of Part One tackles a major area of self-care: over-the-counter products; natural remedies; usage and storage of remedies; the role of your pharmacist; how to be a smart consumer; and children and remedies. The basics that are covered in this part of the book will give you a strong background when it comes to managing those conditions that don't require a doctor's care. They will allow you to feel more confident in your choices of remedies and how to use them.

OVER-THE-COUNTER PRODUCTS (OTCs)

Almost everybody uses over-the-counter products at one time or another. It is estimated that $11 to $12 billion a year is spent on OTCs. There are more than 300,000 OTCs on the market today, although there are only between 750 and 1,000 active ingredients in those thousands and thousands of products. For the average consumer, OTCs are a major part of self-care and a mainstay of the medicine cabinet.

The Definition of OTCs

An over-the-counter product, or OTC, is a medication that you can purchase in a pharmacy or other retail store without first getting a prescription from a physician. Usually, OTCs are relatively inexpensive. They are used to treat minor illnesses and to relieve symptoms. It is estimated that, in the United States, from 70 to 90 percent of illness is self-treated and, for the most part, treated with OTCs.

There is a widespread spectrum of OTCs. These products range from pain relievers and cough syrups to anti-itch creams and antibacterial sprays. For some orally administered products, you have a choice between liquid and pill (capsule/tablet) forms. For some topical OTCs, you can choose from creams or solutions. That's why the drug store aisle can be so intimidating—there are countless bottles and boxes that carry all sorts of promotions and promises. *The Pharmacist's Guide to Over-the-Counter and Natural Remedies* will help you sort through the options and choose one that's right for you. In Part

Two, there are easy-to-find, effective products listed for the treatment of the conditions discussed.

The Benefits and Potential Problems of OTCs

Obviously, OTCs are readily available in your local drug store and can be purchased without a visit to a doctor or clinic. They can help relieve the minor, annoying symptoms of illness that might interfere with daily life if left untreated. In the past, many ineffective and even unsafe OTCs were sold in the United States. However, in the early 1970s, the United States Food and Drug Administration (FDA) began a thorough evaluation of all OTCs on the market. This evaluation is not yet completed. Although OTC products are strictly regulated by the FDA, the system has many critics. While no drug is 100-percent safe, most OTCs are safe and effective when used as directed. The evaluation of these products is ongoing.

There are other benefits to using OTCs, as well. For example, consumers receive far more written information about OTC products from the manufacturers than they receive from the companies who make prescription drugs. Through package inserts and detailed labels, consumers are given specific information about proper use, dosage, side effects, and other important subjects. This allows the purchaser to make informed decisions.

However, an OTC remedy can sometimes prove to be a double-edged sword. While it can quickly bring relief from troubling symptoms, your self-diagnosis may not be correct. The OTC may suppress symptoms of a more serious illness that then remains undiagnosed and, therefore, urgently needed treatment may be delayed. This can lead to serious health consequences. So there is always a risk involved when even the most educated of consumers makes a self-diagnosis and devises a treatment plan.

Too often, consumers get most of their information about OTCs from advertising. Ads often contain claims that, while not untrue, are not *entirely* true either. Marketing ploys designed to gain a large market share or to develop brand loyalty for a particular OTC can lead to exaggerated or misleading claims for products. The consumer who relies on advertising for information about OTCs is not acting in his or her own best interest.

Overusing OTCs can also cause serious problems, particularly with medications that contain combinations of ingredients. Marketing tactics lead some companies to use the same names for products with many different ingredients. For example, a product containing aspirin and caffeine could be labeled by the same name as a product containing just aspirin. Also, many companies sell products with the same ingredients under many different names. As a result, out of ignorance and confusion, a consumer may unwittingly take too much of a particular medication.

Furthermore, OTCs may pose special problems for specific groups of people, such as children and seniors. Children have needs that are different from those of adults. And seniors metabolize drugs differently and cannot be treated with the same regimens as other adults. Also, aging presents special problems in terms of misuse. Seniors, who account for over 25 percent of drug use in the United States, more frequently take several products at the same time, for a number of conditions. In addition, poor vision may lead to trouble reading labels. Older people are also at risk of misusing OTCs if they suffer from any of the following: depression; emotional problems from retirement, the death of a loved one, living alone, or other major life changes; frequent drinking of alcohol; physical pain; or having difficulty asking a doctor or pharmacist questions.

Importantly, the safety associated with over-the-counter products varies considerably for people with pre-existing illnesses for which they may already be taking medication. And women who are pregnant, who think they may be pregnant, or who are nursing must be extremely careful about taking *any* medicinal substances, OTCs included. In such cases, a doctor's guidance is necessary.

Every medication has its adverse effects and no product is 100-percent safe for everybody at all times. But the benefits of OTCs are generally considered to outweigh the risks. The side effects of these products are minimal. However, more and more OTCs now on the market were prescription drugs not long ago (see page 6). Along with the benefits of these products comes the risk of adverse effects that can be more serious than with the less potent OTCs that were available in past years.

Self-care is unavoidable at times, but you must be careful. Studies show that nearly 90 percent of people make mistakes when taking drugs. Over 1 million Americans are injured by such mistakes, many thousands of whom are fatally affected. Lack of information is responsible for about 30 to 50 percent of the consumer mistakes with medicines. The National Pharmaceutical Council, Inc., estimates that the medical costs to remedy drug misuse—for example, treatments for kidney and liver damage—rise into the billions of dollars annually. The most common mistakes people make are: taking incorrect doses; taking doses at the wrong time; forgetting to take doses; and stopping OTC treatment too soon.

When a Prescription Drug Becomes an OTC

Since the late 1970s, nearly 400 drugs that were once available only through a doctor's prescription have become available as over-the-counter products. Every year, patents on prescription drugs expire and these powerful substances become readily available on drug-store shelves. The FDA is taking a "fast track" approach in this area and may be putting the interests of the drug companies ahead of the health of consumers.

Fortunately for the consumer, most of these products have been on the prescription market for nearly twenty years before becoming available over-the-counter. And, because of strict FDA testing requirements, more information on these products is available. Unfortunately, however, these potent medicines are becoming OTCs at a time when economic pressures from HMOs and other third-party payers are interfering with the doctor-patient relationship. As a result, many people no longer have a personal or family physician who knows them well and who can be consulted for advice about the new OTCs. And HMOs are increasingly turning to OTCs in an effort to reduce their own costs; many health plans have to pay for all or most prescription-drug costs, while OTC costs almost always come out of the patient's pocket. So, *more* people are using *more* potent medicines, often with *less* guidance.

Although some health professionals and consumer advocates are concerned about "switching" drugs from prescription to over-the-counter products, these new OTCs are extremely popular with consumers. After all, they can be more effective than traditional products and are usually much less expensive than the prescription versions. Consumers can now self-treat conditions and symptoms such as pain, rashes, and yeast infections with medicines that could previously only be prescribed by a doctor. To treat these conditions and symptoms safely, the consumer needs to be well-informed and *very careful*. When taking potent new OTCs (and all medicines), it is vital for consumers to have written information about the possible side effects and possible interactions with other medicines, herbs, alcohol, tobacco, foods, and dietary supplements.

How to Choose an OTC

When selecting an OTC, you first need to know if the product is recommended, safe, and effective for your condition. Second, you must determine your proper dosage. Third, you need to be aware of any special considerations that apply to using the product. And fourth, you need to know how long it takes for the OTC to start working.

Most people turn to a doctor, nurse, pharmacist, or other health professional for information about medications. Some ask family or friends what OTCs they recommend for minor complaints. Still others try a variety of drugs until they find one that works for them. Of these options, asking a pharmacist for advice is probably the most effective. This medical expert is nearby, wherever you purchase your OTC and natural remedies. In addition, you will be well-served by doing your own homework. Look up your condition in this guide and learn what OTCs are recommended as safe and effective treatments.

The OTC Product's Label

Although Federal law requires that OTC labels include adequate information on proper use, as well as warnings against misuse, about half of all Americans do not read the labels on the OTCs they purchase and do not follow the directions on the containers. *It is extremely important that you read the directions for OTC medications carefully. OTCs are generally safe and effective, but only if you follow the directions and use them as indicated.* Instructions are often found on the product container and/or in a manufacturer's package insert that comes with the product.

The brand or generic name will be the most prominent item on a product's label. The list of ingredients is the next most important information for the consumer. The active ingredient(s) should be listed first, followed by the inactive ingredients. Some OTCs are single-ingredient products, while others are combination-ingredient products.

Obviously, it is easier for consumers to determine exactly what is in single-ingredient products. Furthermore, it is easier to determine the specific conditions that single-ingredient products are recommended to remedy. Combination-ingredient products are more complicated. Therefore, it is especially important that you read the labels of combination-ingredient products with great care. These OTCs may contain ingredients that you do not need to take, that you do not want to take, or to which you may be allergic. Too often, ingredients are combined in products not to produce a better medicine for the consumer, but so that the manufacturer can sell more products. Adding more ingredients to a product is not necessarily done so that the substance can treat a wider range of symptoms, but to create a market share and a brand name for a common product.

The label on the OTC will also provide you with other valuable information, including the name and address of the manufacturer or distributor. And it will list the total amount of the contents, as well as the precise amount of medication in each individual unit of the remedy. Conditions and symptoms for which the product is recommended are addressed. In addition, the expiration date of the product, the batch or lot number, and details about tamper-proof features of the container are provided. Specific directions on how to use the product correctly, including the recommended dosage, can be found on the OTC label. Finally, necessary warnings or cautions about using the product are given.

Self-treatment requires that you take responsibility for learning about the OTCs you use. Reading the label is your first step toward taking good care of yourself. Again, if you decide to use an OTC treatment, it is essential that you meticulously follow the manufacturer's instructions that are found on the label.

NATURAL REMEDIES

The therapeutic use of natural remedies has been practiced around the world throughout history. Natural remedies have remained dominant in Eastern approaches to medicine. Furthermore, in the past few decades, they have been widely used throughout the West, except for in the United States, where synthetic drugs have been dominant since the mid-1900s.

However, American interest in natural remedies has begun to grow rapidly since the early 1990s. As a result, many potent natural treatments have become widely available in drug stores and health-food stores across the United States. And consumer demand has skyrocketed since the mid-1990s, with the passage of the Dietary Supplement Health and Education Act (DSHEA). This act allows companies to carry out more aggressive marketing of dietary supplements.

Now, more and more research is being dedicated to exploring natural methods of prevention and treatment. The current information offered in this guide will enable you to find effective, low-cost natural treatments that are clinically documented and safe.

The Definition of Natural Remedies

The term "natural remedies" covers a wide range of treatments, from herbal supplements—defined as "crude drugs" of vegetable or plant origin, and their common preparations—to vitamins and minerals, to simple lifestyle changes in such areas as diet, relaxation, and exercise. Natural remedies are used to treat common, often chronic disease states that do not require a doctor's monitoring, and to help attain or maintain improved states of health.

There is nothing magical or mystical about natural remedies; they have been used all over the world for thousands of years. Many consider natural remedies—especially herbal remedies—to be *alternative medicine*. However, this is not really accurate. At present, 25 percent of all prescription drugs are derived from plants. Consider Digoxin, for example. Digoxin, a drug that is commonly used to prevent congestive heart failure, is derived from digitalis, which comes from foxglove, a flowering plant that is very common in English gardens. Furthermore, in Germany—a country considered to have a very advanced Western technological society—one out of every four people uses natural remedies as the first line of treatment. Plant medicine is one of the oldest forms of medicine on earth. It could be argued that natural medicine is "mainstream," and that treatment with synthetic chemicals is "alternative."

Herbs and Other Plants

Herbs and other plants are the most recognized form of natural remedies. Their preparations are called *phytomedicinals*, which are made by using various solvents to extract the plants' active ingredients. Herbal remedies are frequently available in several easy-to-use forms, among which are: whole, dried herbs; teas; capsules/tablets; liquid extracts; essential oils; and ointments.

Over 13,000 plants are known to have served as medicines throughout the world. Many of them have been safely applied for centuries. Today, approximately 300 natural remedies are used in the West. Many more are used in the ancient medicine traditions of China, India, and the countries within their spheres of influence, such as Japan. As herbal remedies come into increasing use in American medicine, it is likely that they will be put under the strict scrutiny of well-executed clinical trials. Scientific methodology will be used to verify ancient wisdom, for the benefit of all health consumers.

Choosing an herbal supplement is challenging because there is so much technical information that should be known prior to reading the supplement labels. Refer to the chart on page 24 for information on precautions. Also, every label on an herbal remedy should list an appropriate amount of active constituents. Make sure that the supplement you choose contains this appropriate amount.

It is not sufficient simply to look for the term "standardized" on the label of an herbal supplement. "Standardized extract" gives the impression that the product contains a known quantity and consistent amount of activity in each dose. The problem is that we should not necessarily be looking for the standardization of the herb, but of the active constituents in the herb. For example, if you are purchasing kava kava extract, choose a product that is standardized to 30-percent kavalactones (as kavalactones are the active ingredient) instead of selecting a product that simply states, "standardized kava kava." Another example can be found in garlic supplements; choose tablets that are standardized to allicin potential, as allicin is the active constituent.

Some supplement products, such as Nextract supplements developed by Next Pharmaceuticals, Inc., are specifically formulated to provide consistency—each and every dose contains a specific amount of active constituents—and are also tested for contamination. These qualities are very important to consider. Be sure to select a product made by a reputable manufacturer.

Vitamin and Mineral Supplements

Vitamins and minerals are essential to our health. They take part in every vital function of our bodies, allow us to produce energy, and keep us well. Unfortunately, many people's diets are lacking sufficient amounts of necessary vitamins and minerals. In such cases, supplementation is beneficial.

A central notion behind efforts to provide yourself with healing amounts of vitamins and minerals is *balance*. Too much or too little can harm you. It is also important to keep in mind that vitamins and minerals work *synergistically*, meaning they are more effective in combination rather than if they were to be taken alone.

Our bodies have developed great ability to use vitamins and minerals for health benefits. Supplementation can sometimes restore well-being if you are experiencing certain illnesses. Scurvy is an example of a severe condition that is the result of vitamin-C deficiency. It involves bleeding gums, weakness, and the breaking of blood vessels under the skin. Simply increasing the intake of vitamin C can remedy these terrible symptoms.

Selecting a balanced multivitamin/mineral supplement is challenging because the daily requirement for some minerals is larger than what can be supplied in a single tablet or capsule. If, for example, you want a product that supplies a balanced level of all of the vitamins plus the requirements for calcium and magnesium, you would need to take a daily dosage of four to six tablets. An adequate single tablet would simply be much too large to swallow.

Traditionally, vitamin companies have avoided formulating products that suggest more than a single tablet per daily dosage. This strategy is based upon consumer research that consistently shows that most of us don't like taking a lot of supplements. We'd prefer to have all that we need in a single tablet. But once it is recognized and accepted that one tablet is not enough, there are some helpful guidelines for selecting products that can be used for developing a personalized and balanced supplement program.

First, select a multivitamin product that contains approximately 100 percent of the daily requirement of all vitamins. What can you use as a measuring stick for determining how much of each nutrient you need? Table 1.1 on page 16 offers information about optimal and toxic dosages, and tells you what side effects you may experience.

If the supplement that you are considering contains some minerals, you will need to determine what additional amount you need to get your intake up to 100 percent of the daily requirements for these, as well. It is likely that you will need to take additional mineral supplements in order to reach optimal levels.

Importantly, determine how much additional calcium you need beyond what is being provided

Table 1.1. Vitamin and Mineral Intakes

Nutrient	Suggested Dose	Toxic Dose
Vitamin A	10,000–35,000 IU	100,000–500,000 IU

Comments: Chronic ingestion of even the lesser toxic amount can cause fatigue, headache, nausea, vomiting, vertigo, blurred vision, incoordination of the muscles, and loss of body hair. If supplementation is stopped, the symptoms will terminate. A single extremely high dose can cause acute, although reversible effects. Pregnant women should not take more than 8,000 IU daily.

Beta-carotene	10–30 mg	None determined

Comments: High intakes are not associated with any toxicity symptoms. The only possible side effect is hypercarotenemia (harmless yellowing of the skin).

Vitamin B_1 (Thiamin)	5–10 mg	None determined

Comments: Considered generally safe at all intake levels because the kidneys remove excess amounts.

Vitamin B_2 (Riboflavin)	6–15 mg	None determined

Comments: No reported toxic effects.

Vitamin B_3 (Niacin)	25–100 mg	300–600 mg

Comments: Toxicity symptoms include headache, nausea, and skin blotching (niacinamide form). Flushing, rashes, tingling (nicotinic acid form) and itching can occur. Doses exceeding 2,500 mg daily can cause liver damage and glucose intolerance.

Vitamin B_6 (Pyridoxine)	2 mg	250–1,000 mg

Comments: Prolonged high doses can cause reversible nerve damage.

Vitamin B_{12} (Cobalamin)	4 mcg	None determined

Comments: No reported toxic effects.

Nutrient	Suggested Dose	Toxic Dose
Vitamin C	250–1,000 mg	None determined

Comments: Daily doses of 5,000+ mg can cause loose stools and gas. Some research reveals that doses as high as 10,000 mg daily are not harmful. Yet, doses as low as 1,000 to 2,000 mg might contribute to kidney stones, interactions between minerals, impaired immune function, and withdrawal symptoms. If you have kidney problems, see your physician for supplementation guidelines.

Vitamin D	200–400 IU	> 1,000 IU

Comments: Toxicity symptoms include nausea, vomiting, loss of appetite, dry mouth, headache, and dizziness. Hypercalcemia—high blood-calcium levels—can occur and result in irreversible calcium deposits in the soft tissues and organs.

Vitamin E	50–400 IU	> 1,200 IU

Comments: Start with a lower dose and increase gradually. Safe, even when long-term high doses are taken. Individuals on anticoagulants should avoid doses above 400 IU. Very high doses (in excess of 1,200 IU) can cause nausea, diarrhea, headaches, heart palpitations, flatulence, and fainting. Symptoms disappear when supplementation is reduced.

Calcium	1,000–1,500 mg	3,000–8,000 mg

Comments: If too much calcium builds up in the body, numerous adverse symptoms, including nausea, vomiting, high blood pressure, diarrhea, constipation, and milk-alkali syndrome can occur.

Chromium	200 mcg	None determined

Comments: No reported toxic effects.

Copper	2 mg	None determined

Comments: If too much is taken, nausea, vomiting, headache, and jaundice can occur.

Folacin	400 mcg	None determined

Comments: While there are no reported toxic effects, some women are at risk for low zinc when suplementing with folacin. Also, be sure to take vitamin B_{12} with folacin, as well.

Nutrient	Suggested Dose	Toxic Dose
Pantothenic Acid	10 mg	10,000–50,000 mg

Comments: While generally safe at high doses, diarrhea and water retention may occur.

Nutrient	Suggested Dose	Toxic Dose
Iron	10 mg (males and postmenopausal females) 20 mg (premenopausal females)	18 mg or more

Comments: Constipation and stomach upset can occur. Doses above 100 mg daily can result in abdominal pain, fatigue, weight loss, and possibly heart disease.

Nutrient	Suggested Dose	Toxic Dose
Magnesium	400–600 mg	> 1,000 mg

Comments: Diarrhea, low blood pressure, and nausea can result from toxic dosages.

Nutrient	Suggested Dose	Toxic Dose
Selenium	200 mcg	800–3,000 mg

Comments: Brittle hair and fingernails, dizziness, fatigue, nausea, diarrhea, and liver disease can occur with toxic doses.

Nutrient	Suggested Dose	Toxic Dose
Zinc	15–35 mg	50–150 mg

Comments: Toxicity symptoms include impaired copper absorption, lowered HDL-cholesterol (or "good" cholesterol), impaired immune response, dizziness, vomiting, gastrointestinal problems, and anemia.

by your diet and your supplement. Most adults should target a total of between 1,200 and 1,500 mg of calcium per day. If you do not drink milk and if you don't eat many dairy products, consider supplementing with a calcium product that can supply 1,200 mg daily. This may require taking three or four calcium tablets, spread out over the day. If you consume a moderate amount of dairy, you may only need 600 mg of additional calcium from a supplement.

Instead of just supplementing with calcium alone, look for a complete multimineral formula that, in four to six tablets, supplies the following: 100 percent of the daily requirements for calcium and magnesium; 200 mcg of selenium; 200 mcg of chromium; and a broad range of other minerals. This strategy works fine if you do not eat or drink dairy products. But if you are a moderate to heavy dairy consumer, your best strategy would be to aim for a supplement containing up to 100 percent of the daily requirements of magnesium, chromium, and selenium. Then you can find calcium and magnesium combined in a separate product, sometimes along with zinc. You may find that the most flexible combination is to find a good multivitamin formula with some minerals, and then simply add the calcium/magnesium/zinc supplement according to your needs.

Next, look at the antioxidant levels. The basic antioxidant vitamins are A, C, and E. You probably will get enough vitamin A in your multivitamin, but you will need to increase your C and E if you want to supplement at levels shown to decrease the risk of heart disease and some types of cancer. Consider taking a total daily vitamin-C intake of up to 1,000 to 3,000 mg, and a total daily vitamin-E intake of up to 400 IU. Other antioxidants to consider are grape-seed extract, green tea extract (or simply green tea), lutein, alpha lipoic acid, and lycopene.

Nutrient needs can increase according to an individual's specific life situation. For example, people on long-term medication and individuals under chronic stress often have greater nutrient needs. In addition, oral contraceptives increase vitamin B_6 requirements for women. Smokers need a greater intake of vitamin C. Pregnant and lactating women have increased nutritional needs, as do adolescents. The best way to determine your daily needs is to have a nutritionist assess your personal situation.

Natural Food Supplements

In addition to vitamin/mineral supplements, you can enhance your health with natural food supplements. These are foods or food components that provide special health benefits. For example, garlic contains substances that can lower blood pressure, reduce the risk of clots, fight infection, lower blood cholesterol levels, combat fungal infections, and more. Garlic supplements can come in very handy when you are treating a minor condition. But it is also a wise prevention tactic to include garlic, as a food, in your diet.

Another example of a food supplement is alfalfa. This plant contains chlorophyll and is nutrient-rich. It has calcium, magnesium, potassium, phosphorus, and every vitamin. Alfalfa is a healthy addition to salads, or you can take liquid alfalfa extract.

A final example is fish oils, which provide omega-3 fatty acids. Omega-3s are *essential* fatty acids that take part in many functions, including the healthy maintenance of the cell membranes and the enhancement of immunity. Our bodies cannot produce essential fatty acids on their own. A good balance of fatty acids is critical to our health, and we must attain it through proper diet and supplementation.

Five-A-Day Diet

Healthy dietary decisions are included under the category of natural remedies. It is critically important to eat a balanced diet that includes fresh fruits and vegetables. *Aim to consume at least five servings of both fruits and vegetables per day.* This should be part of a diet consisting mostly of whole foods that do not require preservatives and have not lost their nutrients through processing.

The average American diet includes too much saturated fat, total fat, sugar, cholesterol, protein, and salt. It lacks adequate fiber, complex carbohydrates, fruits, vegetables, vitamins, and minerals. Many Americans go through the entire day without eating one piece of fruit or one whole vegetable. Avoiding these natural foods will only result in deficiencies that, in the end, lead to chronic ailments.

American women's diets are typically low in the nutrients that prevent osteoporosis and anemia, among which are calcium and iron. American men often possess low levels of magnesium, and this deficiency is linked with the increased risk of high

Figure 1.1. USDA Food Guide Pyramid

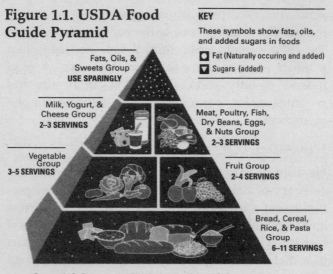

KEY

These symbols show fats, oils, and added sugars in foods

⬤ Fat (Naturally occuring and added)

▼ Sugars (added)

Fats, Oils, & Sweets Group
USE SPARINGLY

Milk, Yogurt, & Cheese Group
2–3 SERVINGS

Meat, Poultry, Fish, Dry Beans, Eggs, & Nuts Group
2–3 SERVINGS

Vegetable Group
3–5 SERVINGS

Fruit Group
2–4 SERVINGS

Bread, Cereal, Rice, & Pasta Group
6–11 SERVINGS

Source: U.S. Department of Agriculture and the U.S. Department of Health and Human Services.

blood pressure and heart attack. In organizing your daily diet, it is helpful to follow some basic guidelines. The U.S. Department of Agriculture has provided the Food Guide Pyramid, which categorizes foods into general groups and, for each, suggests the daily number of servings that you should eat (see Figure 1.1, above). Just keep in mind that, when it comes to fruits and vegetables, we strongly suggest "five a day."

The Benefits and Potential Problems of Natural Remedies

The vast experience with natural remedies over

millennia shows that many are safe and nontoxic, especially when used for minor ailments. Because natural remedies do not pack the short-term punch of synthetic drugs, they cause fewer serious side effects. Natural remedies can be used successfully to boost the immune system, relieve anxiety, and increase energy.

In general, natural remedies are useful for treating chronic problems over a long period of time. But because they are usually less potent than synthetic drugs, natural remedies may be less effective in treating many acute health problems. Furthermore, caution should be exercised when using any substance, and especially exotic natural remedies. The judgment of the effectiveness of lesser-known remedies is based on observation and experience, not on Western scientific clinical testing. Natural remedies can indeed cure, but, as with OTCs, no substance is 100-percent safe and risk-free at all times. Some natural products contain harmful ingredients.

Natural remedies can cause problems if misused or if used in combination with other natural remedies or with certain OTCs and prescription drugs. See Table 1.2, page 24, for more information. It is a common misconception that because a remedy does not contain synthetic ingredients, it is completely safe. The truth is that any remedy is potent enough to instigate changes in your body and should, therefore, be used as carefully as possible. *Make it a point to discuss natural remedies with a health-care professional.* Pharmacists, herbalists,

Table 1.2. Fifty Common Herbs and Their

HERB	INTERACTIONS & PRECAUTIONS
ALOE—*Aloe vera, Aloe barbadensis, Aloe capensis* (Curacao aloe, Cape aloe)—Aloe vera gel comes from either the juice of the inner tissue or the pulverized whole leaf. Aloe latex comes from just under the outer skin of the leaf. (6,14,15)	Topical use of gel—No side effects reported. Oral use of latex products—Can cause abdominal cramping, diarrhea, electrolyte imbalance, and hypokalemia. May potentiate toxicity of cardiac glycosides and thiazide diuretics. Contraindicated in pregnancy (reflex stimulation of uterine musculature). (5,14)
ASTRAGALUS—see Tragacanth	
BEARBERRY (Uva-Ursi)—*Arctostaphylos uva-ursi* (kinnikinnik, hogberry, manzanita)—arbutin is hydrolyzed to hydroquinone in the GI Hydroquinone is released in the urinary tract. (6,15,16)	May cause nausea and vomiting. Urine must be alkaline to release free hydroquinone. Bearberry is inactivated by urinary acidifiers (i.e. cranberry juice). Taking 6–8 g of sodium bicarbonate per day will alkalinize the urine, but not recommended for more than a few days. (5,6,16)
BIRCH LEAF—*Betula verrucosa, Betula pubescens.* (22)	No side effects reported in the literature. Contraindicated with impaired cardiac or renal function. (5)
BLACK COHOSH—*Cimicifuga racemosa* (baneberry, bugbane, bugwort, black snakeroot, squawroot, rattle root, Rernifemin)—not the same as blue cohosh, a potentially toxic plant. (6,15,22,24,25)	May affect the hypothalamus-pituitary system. Contraindicated during pregnancy and lactation. May cause GI disturbances and hypotension. (6,15)
CAPSICUM—*Capsicum frutescens, Capsicum annum* (Capsaicin, Cayenne pepper, Chili pepper, Red pepper, African chilies, Tabasco pepper). (14,15,22)	Can cause local burning sensation. Contamination of hands can transfer to eyes and mucous membranes—wash thoroughly. (22)

* These are not FDA-approved uses. Caution is advised before using or recommending any of these herbs for these purposes.

Potential Interactions With Regular Drugs

USE*	TRADITIONAL DOSING**
Aloe vera gel products used topically are generally shown to be effective for promotion of wound healing and for treatment of burns and frostbite. Preliminary studies show aloe vera gel taken orally may enhance the immune system and has promise for AIDS patients. Aloe latex products are strong cathartics and are rarely recommended. (6,14,22,27)	Topical use—Apply gel as needed. Ingredients deteriorate, so use fresh product for best results. Oral use of aloe latex—Adult daily dose is 0.05–0.2 g of powdered aloe or dry extract. May color the urine red. (5,14)
Used as a urinary tract antibacterial and astringent. Not effective in weight loss products (used as a diuretic). (5,6,16)	Adult mean daily dose is 10 g powdered drug (400–700 mg arbutin) macerated overnight in 150 mL of cold water.*** Maximum effect obtained 3–4 hrs after ingestion. Do not use for more than 1 wk. Urine may appear green. (5,6,15)
Shown to be diuretic in animals. (5,22)	Dose is 2–3 g in boiling water—steep for 10–15 min, strain—take several times per day. Maintain high fluid intake. (5)
Shown to decrease luteinizing hormone (LH). Decreases hot flashes. Used to treat premenstrual discomfort and dysmenorrhea. (6,22)	Adult daily dose is 40–200 mg taken for no more than 6 months. Maximum effect may not be seen for up to 4 wks. (6,22)
Topical use depletes "substance P" and decreases the perception of pain. Shown to be effective for post-herpetic (shingles), trigeminal, and diabetic neuralgia. (22)	Maximum effect seen after applying 4–5 times per day for at least 4 wks; however some effect can occur within 3 days. Pain may initially increase as "substance P" is released before depletion. (15,22)

** In most cases, optimum doses have not been determined through adequate clinical trials. These dosages are representative of traditional use.

*** Cold water maceration reduces tannins.

HERB	INTERACTIONS & PRECAUTIONS
CASCARA—*Rhamnus purshiana* (*Cascara sagrada*, Bitter bark, Chittem bark, Sacred bark)—Buckthorn (Rhamnus frangula) is a different plant but with similar activities. (15)	Don't take if pregnant or lactating. Fresh bark can cause severe vomiting (must be stored for 1 yr or be heat treated). Misuse can deposit pigment in the intestinal mucosa (pseudomelanosis coli), can cause loss of electrolytes and hypokalemia and may potentiate toxicity of cardiac glycosides and thiazide diuretics.
CAT'S CLAW—*Uncaria tomentosa, Uncaria guianensis* (Una de gato). (15)	No reports of toxicity in the literature.
CHAMOMILE—*Matricaria recutita* (German or Hungarian)—despite at least 10 names, all are the same plant. *Chamaemelum nobile* (Roman) is different plant but has similar constituents. (6,16,22)	Rarely, may cause an allergic reaction. Eating large quantities of dried flower heads can cause vomiting. (15)
CHASTE TREE BERRY—*Vitex agnus-castus.* (6)	Rarely, causes GI disturbances, itching. May activate the pituitary, resulting in early onset of menstruation after delivery. May interfere with dopamine-receptor antagonists (animal studies). (5,15)
CRANBERRY—*Vaccinium macrocarpon.* (6)	Overuse (3–4 L juice per day) can cause diarrhea. (15)
DONG QUAI—*Angelica polymorpha, Angelica dahurica, Angelica atropurpurea*	Contraindicated in pregnancy. Has potential to cause photodermatitis. Essential oil contains safrole, a

* These are not FDA-approved uses. Caution is advised before using or recommending any of these herbs for these purposes.

USE*	TRADITIONAL DOSING**
Shown to be a stimulant laxative. (15,22)	Average daily adult dose is 1 g ($\frac{1}{2}$ tsp, 20 to 160 mg of cascara derivatives) in 150 mL of boiling water, strain. Can be taken in the morning and before bedtime. Effects are seen in 6–8 hrs. Should only be taken for a few days. Tea is bitter. (5,15)
Efficacy is anecdotal. An alkaloid constituent has been shown to be hypotensive. Other alkaloids are being studied individually. (15,19)	The root has less activity than the inner bark. No dose determined. (15)
Has antispasmodic, anti-inflammatory (GI tract), anti-microbial activity. Used orally to treat peptic ulcers, spasms of the GI, and inflammation of the mouth and gums. Topically used to treat mucous membrane inflammation, eczema, and to promote wound-healing. (6,22)	Adult dose is 3 g dried flower heads (about 1 heaping tbsp) in 250 mL hot water, steep 10–15 min, strain. Taken 3–4 times daily, between meals. Benefit may be cumulative. Commercial products are frequently adulterated, so best to purchase flower heads. (6,22,23)
Inhibits prolactin release by binding dopamine receptors. Results in increase in lactation. Shown to be effective treatment for menstrual disorders (PMS, mastalgia, menopausal symptoms) by increasing progesterone in relation to estrogen. (6,15)	Adult daily dose is 20 mg of the crude fruit (as extract), or 30–40 mg of the fruits in cold water, then heated to boiling. An infusion tea (boiling water poured over drug) may have less anti-inflammatory activity. (5)
Used to prevent urinary tract infection (UTI). Produces acid urine which prevents microorganisms from attaching to urinary tract. It also reduces urinary odor by retarding the degradation of urine by *E. coli*. (6,15,20,22)	Adult prophylactic dose is 90 mL (45 g fresh berries) daily. Dose to treat UTI is 360–960 mL, daily. Maximum tolerated is 4 L. (6,15,22)
Used to stimulate normal menstrual flow and prevent cramping. Effectiveness controversial. Still	Benefit not worth the risk. Not recommended for use. (15)

** In most cases, optimum doses have not been determined through adequate clinical trials. These dosages are representative of traditional use.

HERB	INTERACTIONS & PRECAUTIONS
(tang-kuei, Dang-gui, Chinese Angelica). (15)	carcinogen. (15)
ECHINACEA—*Echinacea angustifolia, Echinacea pallida*—Purple cone flower (*Echinacea purpurea*) is a different species with same properties. (6,15,16,22)	Possibly becomes immunosuppressive with continuous use (6–8 wks). Contraindicated in patients with autoimmune diseases. Echinacea injections are not recommended (can cause chills, fever, nausea, vomiting, allergies). (5,6,15)
ELEUTHERA—see Siberian Ginseng	
EPHEDRA—see Ma Huang	
FEVERFEW—*Tanacetum parthenium.* (6)	May have GI effects. Fresh leaves can cause mouth ulceration. Do not use in pregnancy (may stimulate menstruation) or during lactation, or in children under 2 yrs. May interact with anticoagulants to increase bleeding. (6,15,16,22)
GARLIC—*Allium sativum*—when the cells of the bulb are crushed, alliin is converted to allicin (responsible for many of garlic's effects and its odor). (6,15)	Shown to inhibit platelet aggregation. May interact with anticoagulants. Reduces blood sugar so may affect glucose control. Rarely, causes allergic reactions. Heat and acid destroy ingredients responsible for cholesterol lowering, so enteric-coated products show best results. (6,15,23)
GINGER—*Zingiber officinale* (6)	Inhibits thromboxane synthetase (platelet aggregation inducer) and is a prostacyclin agonist (inhibitor of platelet aggregation)—may result in prolonged bleeding time. Avoid during pregnancy (controversial) and during times in chemotherapy or after surgery when bleeding is a concern. (6,22)
GINKGO—*Ginkgo biloba.* (6)	Ginkgolide is a selective antagonist of platelet aggregation. Case report of

* These are not FDA-approved uses. Caution is advised before using or recommending any of these herbs for these purposes.

USE*	TRADITIONAL DOSING**
being studied for this and other uses. (15)	
Proven effective for prophylaxis and treatment of cold and flu symptoms. May work by stimulating the production of phagocytes. (6,13,15,16)	Concentrations of chemical constituents in commercial products vary. Maximum adult daily dose is 6–9 mL of expressed fresh juice, or 1.5–7.5 mL of tincture (preferred since not all constituents are water soluble), or 2–5 g of dried root used for no more than 6–8 wks. (5,6,15,22)
Shown to be effective for prophylaxis and treatment of migraine. Has spasmolytic effects on cerebral vessels. Used to treat fevers and menstrual problems. Is not effective for treating rheumatoid arthritis. (6,15,16,22)	Concentrations of chemical constituents in commercial products vary. Adult dose is 125 mg dried leaves (parthenolide content no less than 0.2%) 1–2 times daily. (6,16,22,23)
Shown to be effective for reducing cholesterol, LDL, and triglycerides, and for raising HDL. May have antibacterial, antifungal, antithrombotic, hypotensive, hypoglycemic, antihyperlipidemic, anti-inflammatory, and anticancer activity. (6,13,22)	Concentrations of chemical constituents in commercial products vary. Adult daily dose is 4–12 mg of alliin (2–5 mg of allicin), or 0.4–12 g of dried powder, or 2–5 g of fresh bulb. Decrease in cholesterol may take 8–16 wks, hypotensive effects 1–6 months. (6,13,23)
Shown to be effective for treatment of motion sickness and nausea. Shown to be an effective anti-inflammatory for treatment of arthritis. Positive inotropic effect on heart tissue being studied. (3,6,15,23)	Adult dose is 1 g 30 min prior to travel, then 0.5–1 every 4 hrs (maximum daily dose is 2–4 g). Dose used prior to cancer chemotherapy is 1 g. (3,6,23)
Dilates arteries, capillaries and veins. Used to increase peripheral	Adult dose is 60–80 mg of standardized leaf extract (24%

** In most cases, optimum doses have not been determined through adequate clinical trials. These dosages are representative of traditional use.

HERB	INTERACTIONS & PRECAUTIONS
	spontaneous bleeding from the iris when given with aspirin and of a subdural hematoma with chronic use. May cause minor GI disturbances. Rarely, causes headache, dizziness, vertigo. (6,7,17,18)
GINSENG—*Panax ginseng* (Korean ginseng), *Panax quinquefolium* (American ginseng)—Siberian ginseng is a different species (see separate listing). (6)	Nervousness and excitation can occur for first few days of intake. Overuse can cause headache, insomnia, and palpitations. Use caution in patients with hypertension. Case report of an interaction between ginseng and furosemide (decreased diuretic effect) resulting in hospitalization (probably caused by germanium contamination). Estrogenic effects have caused vaginal bleeding, breast nodules. (3,4,9,15)
GOLDENROD—*Solidago virgaurea, Solidago serotina, Solidago gigantea, Solidago canadensis.* (6)	Rarely, causes allergies. (6)
GOLDENSEAL—*Hydrastis canadensis.* (6)	Contraindicated during pregnancy. High doses may cause nausea, vomiting, diarrhea, CNS stimulation, and respiratory failure. (6,15)
GOTU KOLA—*Centella asiatica*—Titrated extract of *C. asiatica* (TECA)—do not confuse with Kolanut, a different plant with different action. (5)	Contact dermatitis. Large doses can be sedating. (15)
GRAPESEED EXTRACT—*Vitis vinifera*—Pinebark extract *(Pinus maritima, Pinus nigra)* contains the same chemical	No adverse reactions reported.

* These are not FDA-approved uses. Caution is advised before using or recommending any of these herbs for these purposes.

USE*	TRADITIONAL DOSING**
blood flow. Shown to improve intermittent claudication. Used to treat varicosity, cerebral vascular insufficiency, dementia, tinnitus, vertigo, SSRI-induced sexual dysfunction. (6,14,11)	flavone glycosides and 6% terpenes) taken 2–3 times daily. Effects can take from 1–2 months to appear. (3,6,14,22)
Effectiveness not adequately documented. Used prophylactically as an adaptogen to "normalize" the body and provide resistance to stress. May lower blood cholesterol and improve LDL & HDL ratios. Some ingredients raise BP and some lower BP. Not effective as an aphrodisiac. (5,6)	Contents of commercial products vary. Frequently mislabeled or adulterated. Roots must be a minimum of 3 yrs old to be most effective. Adult dose is 1–2 g of root daily, or 100–300 mg of extract (standardized to contain 7% ginsenosides) 3 times daily taken for 3–4 wks. Maximum effects, if any, appear over long term. (6,15,23)
Used for prevention and treatment of urinary tract inflammation, urinary calculi, and kidney stones. (6)	Adult dose is 3–5 g of the herb in 240 mL, boiling water, steep for 15 min, strain. Mean daily dose is 6–12 g. (5,6)
Efficacy not substantiated by clinical studies. Used traditionally to treat mucosal inflammation and gastritis. Does not mask urine drug screens. (6,14,22)	Adult dose is 0.5–1 g of the dried root, or 2–4 mL of tincture, 3 times daily. A tea made from up to 6 g in 240 mL of water has been suggested for mouth sores. Plants take 3–4 yrs to grow to marketability. (6,22)
Shown topically to promote wound healing, including bladder lesions. Topical use may clear psoriasis. Being investigated for anticancer (in-vitro), antihypertensive, and antifertility effects. (15)	Apply topically daily. Oral adult daily dose is 600 mg powdered leaf.
Used as an antioxidant to treat hypoxia from atherosclerosis, inflammation, cardiac, or cerebral infarction. Prevention of connec-	Adult dose of 75–300 mg daily for 3 wks, then 40–80 mg daily maintenance dose. (6)

** In most cases, optimum doses have not been determined through adequate clinical trials. These dosages are representative of traditional use.

HERB	INTERACTIONS & PRECAUTIONS
constituents but is trade-marked "pycnogenol." (6,15)	
GUARANA—*Paullinia cupana* (Zoom)—Contains caffeine 2.5–5% (coffee seed contains 1–2%). (5,15,16)	May cause hypertension and excess stimulation. Extracts have inhibited platelet aggregation. (15)
HAWTHORN—*Crataegus laevigata, Crataegus monogyna, Crataegus pinnatifida.* (7)	High doses cause CNS depression and hypotension. May interact with blood pressure or heart medications. (15)
HOPS—*Humulus lupulus*—related to marijuana. (15)	Contact dermatitis. (15)
HOREHOUND—*Marrubium vulgare.* (6)	No side effects reported in humans. Large doses may produce cardiac irregularities. (22)
HORSE CHESTNUT—*Aesculus hippocastanum* (buckeye)—not the same as the sweet chestnut (*Castanea sativa*) used for cooking. (5,15)	Whole horse chestnuts are toxic. The principal toxin is aesculin. Coumarin-like constituents may interfere with anticoagulants. *Venastat,* standard-ized horse chestnut seed extract, does not contain aesculin. (5) (26)
KAVA-KAVA—*Piper methylsticum.* (15)	High doses can cause muscle weakness. Chronic ingestion causes reversible skin discoloration and eye disturbances. Potentiates alcohol and other CNS depressants. Contraindicated in pregnancy, lactation, endogenous depression. (15,21)
KOLANUT—*Cola nitida* (Cola, Kola)—contains up to 3.5% caffeine (coffee seed contains 1–2%). (16,22)	Cardiac effects (tachyphylaxis) prevent use as a diuretic. (22)

* These are not FDA-approved uses. Caution is advised before using or recommending any of these herbs for these purposes.

USE*	TRADITIONAL DOSING**
tive tissue breakdown is not clinically proven. (6,15)	
An effective CNS stimulant. Used to treat drowsiness and to potentiate analgesics. (6,15,16)	Adult daily dose of caffeine is 100–200 mg. (7)
Used to treat heart disease, angina, sleep disorders. Shown to dilate coronary blood vessels. (15)	Minimum daily adult dose is listed as 5 mg flavone (hyperoside), 10 mg total flavonoids, or 5 mg oligomeric procyanidins (epicatechin)—or a tea of 3–4 g of dried herb taken in 1 g doses 2–3 times daily. (5,6)
May have sedative effects, although evidence is conflicting. Active ingredients increase when herb is stored 1–2 yrs. Does not have estrogenic activity. (5,15,22)	Tea made from .5 g (1–2 tsp) in boiling water, steep for 5–10 min, strain. Taken 2–3 times daily and before bedtime. (5)
Controversial use as expectorant, antitussive, cough suppressant, digestive aid, appetite stimulant. Hypoglycemic in rabbits. (6,15)	Adult dose is 2 g (2 heaping tsp) of dried cut herb in 240 mL of boiling water. Taken 3–5 times per day (up to 0.75–1 L per day). (6,22)
Used traditionally to treat varicose veins and other venous insufficiencies.	High risk/benefit ratio. Not recommended for self-preparation. Dose of *Venastat,* a commercially prepared horse chestnut seed extract, is 1 capsule 2 times daily.
CNS depressant effects and euphoria. Used for sleep inducement and anxiety reduction. (15,21)	History of ceremonial use. Adult daily dose is 60–120 mg kava pyrones. (21)
Used in beverages for caffeine content. (22)	Used in commercial beverages. (16,22)

** In most cases, optimum doses have not been determined through adequate clinical trials. These dosages are representative of traditional use.

HERB	INTERACTIONS & PRECAUTIONS
LEMON BALM—*Melissa officinalis* (sweet balm). (5,6)	No side effects reported with topical use. Decreased thyrotrophin levels in animals. (5,6)
LICORICE—*Glycyrrhiza glabra, Glycyrrhiza uralensis.* (15)	Considered unsafe. High doses (more than 50 g QD) can cause pseudoaldosteronism resulting in increased blood pressure, water retention, and potassium loss. Contraindicated during pregnancy and in patients with liver disorders, hypokalemia, or who are taking cardiac glycosides. Thiazide diuretics may increase potassium loss. May have estrogen-like effects. (5,6,19)
MA HUANG—*Ephedra sinica, E. intermedia, E. equisetina, E. distachya* (squaw tea, Mormon tea, popotillo, sea grape)—Over 40 species, whose contents vary, some contain alkaloids including ephedrine, pseudoephedrine. (6,16,22)	Misuse has caused deaths. Can cause hypertension, CNS stimulation (nervousness, insomnia, palpitations). Can cause hyperglycemia. Ephedrine can be used to manufacture methamphetamine and methcathinone. (6,15)
MILK THISTLE—*Silybum marianum* (silymarin is a mixture of derivatives found only in the fruit). (5,6)	Few adverse effects. Mild diarrhea, allergic reactions, one report of urticaria. Do not use in decompensated cirrhosis. (6,15)
NETTLE—*Urtica dioica.* (2)	Do not use in patients with impaired cardiac or renal function. Rarely, causes allergic reactions. (5)

---

* These are not FDA-approved uses. Caution is advised before using or recommending any of these herbs for these purposes.

USE*	TRADITIONAL DOSING**
Traditionally used to treat sleep disorders and nervous GI disorders. Proven effective topical treatment for early stages of herpes simplex virus lesions. (6)	Use topically. Tea for oral use made from 1.5–2 g (1–3 tsps) of finely chopped drug. In boiling water, steep for 5–10 min, strain. Take several times per day. (5)
Used to treat peptic ulcers (helps increase prostaglandins). Used as an expectorant. (6)	Use of deglycyrrhizinated licorice (DGL) may allow ulcer healing without major side effects, but results are inconclusive. Do not use licorice longer than 4–6 wks. (6,15,23)
Shown to be effective treatment for bronchial asthma—bronchodilator, vasoconstrictor, reduces bronchial edema. Not shown safe and effective for weight loss, although it is an ingredient in many weight loss products. (6)	Concentration of chemical constituents in commercial products varies. The North and Central American species (*Ephedra nevadensis*—Mormon Tea) contains no alkaloids. Adult dose is 2 g (1 heaping tsp—15–30 mg of ephedrine) in 240 mL boiling water, steep for 10 min. (6,22)
Hepatoprotective and antioxidant. Shown to be useful in treating inflammatory liver disorders and cirrhosis (scavenges free radicals, alters outer liver cell membrane structures, blocks binding sites, helps activate the liver's regenerative capacity). Shown to protect liver against damage from toxins. (6,22)	Adult dose of seeds is 12–15 g per day (200–240 mg of silymarin). Tea not an effective dosage form. (6,22)
Fresh sap has shown a mild diuretic effect. Roots may relieve benign prostatic hyperplasia (BPH) symptoms. Root and leaves are being studied to reduce inflammation, interact with androgen transport, and stimulate the immune system.	Adult daily dose of root for BPH is 4–6 g. Tea is made from 4 g (3–4 tsp) herb in hot water, steep 10 min, strain. Taken 3–4 times daily. (5)

** In most cases, optimum doses have not been determined through adequate clinical trials. These dosages are representative of traditional use.

HERB	INTERACTIONS & PRECAUTIONS
PASSION FLOWER—*Passiflora incarnata* (Maypop). (5)	No adverse reactions reported. May have some MAOI activity. (15)
PAU D'ARCO—*Lapacho colorado, Tabebuia avellanedae* (Taheebo, Trumpet bush, lapacho). (15)	Active ingredients shown to be toxic to humans. Has anticoagulant effects. Causes nausea, vomiting, dizziness. (8,15,22)
PEPPERMINT—*Mentha x piperita.* (6,15)	Oil may irritate mucous membranes. Do not use in infants or children. Tea from leaves may cause laryngeal and bronchial spasms in small children. Overuse leads to heartburn and relaxation of the lower esophageal sphincter. May worsen hiatal hernia symptoms. May cause allergic reactions, contact dermatitis. (6,15)
PRIMROSE, EVENING—*Oenothera biennis.* (15)	Studies have shown no adverse reactions or toxicity. (15)
PSYLLIUM—*Plantago arenaria, Plantago psyllium, Plantago indica, Plantago ovata* (Plantain, Plantago). (6,16)	Rarely, causes allergic reaction (anaphylaxis). May interfere with the absorption of other drugs. Wait 30–60 minutes between dosing. Bezoars (GI blockage) may form if not taken with enough fluid. (6,15)
PUMPKIN SEEDS—*Cucurbitae peponis.* (5,13)	No adverse effects reported. (5)

* These are not FDA-approved uses. Caution is advised before using or recommending any of these herbs for these purposes.

USE*	TRADITIONAL DOSING**
No clinical evidence for effectiveness of fruit (seed). (13,15,22)	
Used as a sedative, but not supported by clinical trials in humans. (15)	Adult daily dose is a tea of 4–8 g (3–6 tsp) taken in divided doses 2–3 times daily and before bedtime. (5,22)
Said to be anticancer agent and anti-inflammatory, but evidence is inconclusive. The National Cancer Institute found no significant antineoplastic effects. (15,22)	High risk, little or no benefit. Not recommended for use.
Shown to decrease muscle spasms of the GI tract. Used to treat abdominal pain. Oil used as a flavoring agent and a digestive aid. Enteric-coated capsules used to treat irritable bowel syndrome (IBS). (6,15)	Tea is made from 1–1.5 g (1 tbsp) leaves in 160 mL of boiling water, steep for up to 10 min, taken 3–4 times daily. Dose of Peppermint Spirit (10% oil and 1% leaf extract) is 1 mL (20 drops) taken with water. (6,22)
Shown to lower serum cholesterol. Shown to improve atopic eczema. Used as a GLA (gammalinoleic acid) supplement (can be converted to the prostaglandin precursor DGLA). Being studied for a variety of conditions. (15)	Adult daily dose for GLA supplementation is 0.6–6 g. Adult dose for atopic eczema is 1 g 2 times daily. (6)
Shown useful as a bulk-forming laxative for constipation, irritable bowel syndrome (IBS), and for lowering cholesterol and LDL levels. (6,15)	Dose is 7.5–10 g plus at least 150 mL water for each 5 g of drug. Take 30–60 min after a meal. Component in seeds may be nephrotoxic so commercial products are preferable. (6,15)
Used to increase urination in patients with BPH, but not substantiated by clinical trials. (5,13)	Maximum adult dose is 15–30 g (1–2 heaping tbsp) taken with fluid 2 times daily. Efficacy may not be seen for weeks or months. (5)

** In most cases, optimum doses have not been determined through adequate clinical trials. These dosages are representative of traditional use.

HERB	INTERACTIONS & PRECAUTIONS
PYCNOGENOL—see Grape-seed Extract	
ST. JOHN'S WORT—*Hypericum perforatum*—the active ingredient, hypericin, has been given an IND and is being studied. (2,6,15)	May have monoamine oxidase inhibitor (MAOI) activity. May cause photodermatitis. (2,5,6) Is thought to increase serotonin levels. Don't take with Prozac or other antidepressants. (1)
SARSAPARILLA—*Smilax aristolochiaefolia* (Mexican), *Smilax febrifuga* (Ecuadorian), *Smilax regilii* (Honduras)—unrelated to American or Wild Sarsaparilla (*Aralia nudicaulis*). (12)	Causes irritation of mucous membranes (throat, intestines). May interfere with absorption of simultaneously administered drugs. Increases absorption of digitalis and bismuth, and elimination of hypnotics. (12)
SAW PALMETTO—*Serenoa repens* (sabal, cabbage palm). (6)	Rarely can cause upset stomach, mild headache. High doses can cause diarrhea. Do not use during pregnancy or lactation or in children. Effect on other hormone therapy not known. (15)
SENNA—*Cassia acutifolia, Cassia angustifolia, Senna alexandrina.* (5)	Chronic use can result in electrolyte imbalances and potassium loss. May increase toxicity of cardiac glycosides. May turn urine red. Long term use can cause pigmentation of the colon (pseudomelanosis coli) and reversible finger clubbing. (5,6,15)
SIBERIAN GINSENG—*Eleutherococcus senticosus* (eleuthera)—same family but not the same species or composition as *Panax Ginseng.* (15,22)	No adverse reactions reported. (Toxicity reports have been related to adulterants). May produce aggressive behavior in animals. (22)

* These are not FDA-approved uses. Caution is advised before using or recommending any of these herbs for these purposes.

USE*	TRADITIONAL DOSING**
Shown to be effective for the treatment of mild-to-moderate depression. May have sedative and anti-inflammatory activity. (6,10)	Adult dose being studied is 300 mg 3 times daily for no more than 8 wks. Tea made with 2–4 g (1–2 tsp) in boiling water, steep 5–10 min. Take 1–2 cups 2 times daily. (2,5)
Folk use only—traditionally used to treat syphilis and as a diuretic. Being promoted erroneously for body-building. Does not contain testosterone, nor is it converted to anabolic steroids. (12,22)	Use only as a flavoring agent. (22)
Fruit extract shown to be effective for treatment of benign prostatic hyperplasia (BPH). Effects are on testosterone uptake and availability (no changes in testosterone plasma levels). Also has anti-inflammatory effects. (6,2,15)	Adult dose is 1–2 g of ground, dried fruit daily, or 80 mg of standardized lipoidal extract (85–95% of fatty acids and sterols) 2 times daily. Teas are ineffective (aqueous extracts have little value). (6,23)
Cathartic, used to treat constipation. (More drastic than cascara, but less expensive). (22)	Do not take for more than 1 to 2 wks without consulting a health care professional. Conc. of teas varies, so standardized commercial dosage forms are preferable. Tea can be made from 0.5–2 g (½–1 tsp) soaked in cold water 10–12 hrs, or hot for 10 min. Effects can take 10–12 hrs after ingestion to be seen. (5,6,22)
Use not supported by adequate clinical studies. Not proven to increase endurance. Injectable form being studied to increase levels of immunocompetent cells (T-cells). (15,22)	Frequently mislabeled or adulterated. (22)

** In most cases, optimum doses have not been determined through adequate clinical trials. These dosages are representative of traditional use.

HERB	INTERACTIONS & PRECAUTIONS
SLIPPERY ELM—*Ulmus rubra.* (6,15)	Pollen is allergenic. May cause contact dermatitis. (15)
TEA TREE OIL—*Melaleuca alternifolia* (Melaleuca, Australian Tea Tree). (15)	Rarely, causes allergic reactions or skin irritation. (6)
TRAGACANTH—*Astragalus gummifera.* (15)	Very susceptible to bacterial degradation. (15)
VALERIAN—*Valeriana officinalis*—other species used for other purposes, *Valeriana edulis* (Mexican), *Valeriana wallichii* (Indian). (5,6,16)	May cause increased morning drowsiness. Is not synergistic with alcohol, but has not been studied with opiates or other CNS depressants. (15,23)
WHITE WILLOW—*Salix purpurea, Salixfragilis, Safix daphnoides* contain the most salicin; however, *Salix alba* is also used. (5,6)	May show adverse reactions similar to salicylates. However, not shown to effect platelet function or to interact with anticoagulants. (5,6)
WITCH HAZEL—*Hamamelis virginiana.* (6)	Tannins in 1 g will cause nausea, vomiting, or constipation. Tannins present in oral preparations may cause liver damage. (5,15)
YERBA MATÉ—*flex paraguariensis* (Maté, Paraguay tea)—contains up to 2% caffeine (similar to coffee beans). (15,16)	May cause hypertension, excess stimulation. Heavy use increases risk of esophageal cancer. (15)
YOHIMBE—*Pausinystalia yohimbe* (Yohimbine). (16)	High risk/benefit ratio. Can cause CNS stimulation, hypotension or hypertension, tachycardia, nausea, vomiting, and psychoses. May have MAOI activity. (22)

* These are not FDA-approved uses. Caution is advised before using or recommending any of these herbs for these purposes.

This chart has been reprinted with permission from *Pharmacist's Letter* and *Prescriber's Letter*. References found on page 353. Numbers following information in columns refer to applicable references. The contents of this chart come from Natural Database, which is published by *Pharmacist's Letter/Prescriber's Letter*, P.O. Box 8190, Stockton, CA 95208, Phone: 209–472–2240.

USE*	TRADITIONAL DOSING**
Acts as a demulcent and an emollient to treat sore throats, gastritis, colitis, gastric or duodenal ulcers. (6,15)	Adult dose is 0.5–2 g of powdered bark steeped in 10 parts hot water (5–20 mL). (5)
Bacteriostatic, germicidal. Used to treat boils, abscesses, cuts, abrasions and acne. Other uses not verified. (6,15)	Apply topically. Has been used in concentrations from 0.4–100%. (22)
Used as an emulsifier and thickening agent. Not proven to decrease serum lipids or blood glucose levels. (15)	Maximum viscosity not reached for 24 hrs at room temp. or 8 hrs with high heat, when mixed with water. (15)
Shown to have mild sedative/hypnotic effects. Used to promote sleep; does not decrease night awakenings. (6,15)	Adult dose is 1–3 g (1–3 mL tincture) 1–3 times daily and before bedtime. (5,6,23)
Used as an analgesic. Salicin is converted to salicylic acid. Probably provides a subtherapeutic source. (6,22)	Concentrations of chemical constituents in commercial products vary. Longer to onset and longer acting than salicylic acid. Hard to reach therapeutic dose by using plant alone. (6,22)
Astringent, anti-inflammatory, hemostyptic. Used to treat inflammation of skin and mucous membranes, but efficacy not supported. (6,15)	Apply topically. The steam distilled product does not contain tannins; therefore, activity probably results from alcohol. Not recommended for oral use. (6,15,22)
An effective CNS stimulant. Used to treat drowsiness and to potentiate analgesics. (6,15)	Adult daily dose of caffeine is 100–200 mg. Tea made with 1 tsp leaves in hot water, steep for 5–10 min, strain. (5,6)
Used to treat impotence—has alpha-2-adrenergic blocking activity. (16)	Recommended for use only under the care of a physician.

** In most cases, optimum doses have not been determined through adequate clinical trials. These dosages are representative of traditional use.

The users of this document are cautioned to use their own professional judgment and consult any other appropriate resources prior to making clinical judgments related to topics in this document. We acknowledge Jan Beckwith, PharmD, Director, Idaho Drug Information Service, Idaho State University, Pocatello, ID, for her outstanding work in the creation of this chart for the subscribers of *Pharmacist's Letter* and *Prescriber's Letter*.

nutritionists, and many physicians can help you learn more about specific supplements/remedies and their relationships to other substances.

USAGE AND STORAGE OF REMEDIES

There's a lot more to a remedy than what a commercial promises or what an anecdote teaches. Keep the following guidelines in mind, to ensure that you are taking the necessary precautions and doing everything you can to properly self-manage your condition.

Top Twenty Tips for the Safe Usage of OTCs and Natural Remedies

The following tips are important when you are treating yourself with any remedy. Not all of these rules will apply to every situation.

- Don't take a medication without looking at the container. You may have picked up the wrong OTC by accident. *Read the label carefully and under bright light before using any product.* This is the first, most important step in properly and safely using a remedy.

- Never remove the original labeling.

- Keep all medications in their original containers.

- Learn the generic as well as the brand names of any products you use.

- Know all of the health effects offered by the remedy, including any potential side effects.

- Check the expiration date before using a product. Discard outdated products.

- Take the remedy only as directed, for the suggested duration of treatment. Follow directions carefully.

- Consult a physician if you begin to experience any adverse effects.

- Never take medications or treatments with alcoholic beverages.

- Know what foods, drinks, and other medicines and activities to avoid when taking the remedy. For example, dairy can inactivate some antibiotics, and citrus can prevent the proper absorption of zinc.

- Keep a complete record of the OTCs and natural remedies you are taking.

- Keep a doctor's or pharmacist's written instructions handy, and ask any questions *before* using the remedy.

- Do not crush or split tablets or capsules without consulting a doctor or pharmacist.

- Re-evaluate long-term treatment at regular intervals.

- Never store remedies near dangerous, toxic substances.

- Be observant and look for signs of product

tampering—for example, broken seals; puncture holes; damaged wrappings.

• Never take discolored remedies or remedies that have unusual odors.

• Never take a remedy when you are not alert or when you have impaired vision.

• Never take anyone else's medication.

• If your condition or symptoms persist or worsen, see a physician.

Although you do not necessarily need to consult with a physician before using an OTC or natural remedy, it is very important that you tell your doctor about every remedy you are taking. As discussed previously, some herbal remedies can be dangerous if combined with certain medications. And some prescription drugs and OTCs can cause serious health problems if taken together. In addition, before a surgical procedure, tell the doctor, anesthetist, or dentist about any substances that you are taking, including OTCs and herbs.

Proper Storage of Remedies

Avoid storing your OTCs and natural substances in the bathroom, if possible. Although this is where most Americans keep their medications, it is not good to store these products in damp places. Also, keep your remedies away from heat and direct light. Dampness, heat, and direct light can alter the chemistry of products and render them ineffective.

It is important that you not leave medication in your car too long for the same reasons. Extremes of temperature can damage the products. A dry, dark storage place is best.

If the OTC or natural remedy you purchase has cotton plugs in the container, remove and discard the cotton upon opening the product. Cotton attracts moisture, which can damage the remedy's effectiveness. If the remedy is a liquid, don't store it in the refrigerator unless you are specifically advised to do so by the directions on the label. The cold can damage the liquid, as can inadvertent freezing. Finally, be sure to keep your remedies out of the reach of children.

THE IMPORTANT ROLE OF YOUR PHARMACIST

Your physician may be the most prominent member of your personal health-care team, but your pharmacist may prove to be the most helpful when it comes to OTC products and natural remedies. The pharmacist can explain what a given product is and how it works. He or she can teach you how to take the remedy safely and effectively.

What to Expect From Your Pharmacist

If at all possible, try to purchase all of your medications—OTCs, prescriptions, supplements, and other remedies—from the same pharmacist. This way, your pharmacist can keep accurate records that may prove invaluable to you and your family. If you provide the pharmacist with a medical history that contains information about your current conditions and any medications you are taking, he or she can help you to avoid dangerous drug interactions and serious side effects.

Don't hesitate to ask your pharmacist to give you written instructions and information about the medications you are taking. You should be as informed as possible. A set of clear instructions could make all the difference, especially when you are not feeling well. Last but not least, your pharmacist can be your best guide to current information on the costs of competing OTCs and natural health-care options, to help save you money.

How Your Pharmacist Can Help With Compliance

Pharmacists can be very useful when it comes to *compliance*—that is, taking your medicines properly. Women who take birth control pills are familiar with the "blister pack" marked for each day of the month. This compliance aid helps them to correctly follow the necessary pill schedule for the birth control to be effective.

The National Council of Patient Information and Education in Washington, DC, has a catalog of patient compliance aids from which your pharmacist can order. For example, among the helpful aids available are a container that beeps when it's time to take your medicine, and a bottle cap that counts the number of times it's been opened (letting you know whether you took the day's dosage). Many pharmacies also carry such items as spoons and syringes that hold a specific dose, and convenience containers organized to sort pills according to the meal with which they are to be taken. New products are always coming to the market. Talk to your pharmacist about compliance aids.

How to Select a Pharmacist

Many people do a great deal of research before selecting a physician and a health plan. If you put as much thought and effort into selecting a pharmacist, you will benefit greatly. Try calling the pharmacy you are considering, to see if the pharmacist can be reached easily by phone. It is important to learn the hours that your pharmacy is open each day, and whether it is open nights, weekends, and holidays. From this information, you can determine how available your pharmacist and his or her colleagues will be.

In addition, go to the pharmacy and see if it is possible to speak with the pharmacist privately, away from the other customers. There should be a space that accommodates private conversation. At times, you may want to discuss some topics with the pharmacist in confidence.

Some pharmacies offer special services, such as consumer education, that may be of interest to you and may lead you to choose one pharmacist over another. Pharmacists are increasingly knowledgeable about herbal and other natural products, as well as about OTC remedies and prescription drugs. Choose one in whom you feel confident. A recent survey showed that 94 percent of pharmacists believe complementary medicine is beneficial; 50 percent have educational credits in complementary medicine; 72 percent counsel consumers about natural remedies; and 100 percent report having been asked about natural remedies by consumers.

And here's another pointer: If you are moving to a new location, ask your former pharmacist for a complete set of your records, which you can then give to the pharmacist in your new neighborhood.

HOW TO BE A SMART CONSUMER

When it comes to conditions that do not require a doctor's careful monitoring, both OTCs and natural remedies can offer you quick symptomatic relief and safe treatment. They can save you money as well. Compared to the cost of prescription drugs, most of these products are a bargain. And if you use generic versions of popular OTCs, your savings will be even greater.

The Quality of the Product

As a rule, generic OTCs are as safe and effective as their more expensive brand-name competitors. In fact, many generics are made by the same companies that make the brand-name products. The medications are then sold in bulk to companies that distribute them under a variety of names nationwide.

Advertising is so powerful, pervasive, and effective that many people are convinced that generic

OTCs are inferior to brand-name products. The next time you are in a pharmacy, compare the list of active ingredients on a generic with that on a brand-name OTC. Then compare the price. Don't be surprised if the brand name costs five times or even ten times more than the generic. What does that extra money pay for—a superior product? No, the extra money that comes out of your pocket pays for the manufacturer's advertising campaigns. Smart consumers avoid paying more than necessary by reading the labels carefully.

Advertising also plays a key role regarding natural remedies. Ads will highlight the benefits of a particular brand of product, but they will not tell you all you need to know. The lay person cannot tell from an ad how the ingredients were collected or what standards prevailed in the manufacture of the natural product.

There are no official United States government standards applicable today regarding natural remedies. Some large companies may be more reliable than smaller firms, but this is not always the case. One recent study showed that 60 percent of ginseng capsules/tablets evaluated provided no particular health benefits, and 25 percent actually contained no ginseng at all! It is crucial that the consumer know the reputation of the manufacturer. (See page 13 for more information.)

The Financial Issue

Prices for OTCs and natural remedies vary widely from store to store. A recent survey done by the

Consumer Affairs Department in New York City found that OTC prices can vary by as much as 30 to 40 percent between stores that are only a few blocks from one another. It pays to shop around for the best price you can find. You may not have to go far to achieve significant savings.

In most states, OTCs and natural remedies are not taxable items. However, few people know this—neither customers nor cashiers—and so millions of people wind up paying an extra 8 percent or more for their remedy purchases. It will benefit you to learn the laws regarding OTCs and natural remedies in your part of the country. Since local tax laws vary greatly and change over the years, it is wise to check with your local consumer affairs bureau to find out what laws apply to your location.

Awareness of Your Particular Needs

Being a smart consumer involves more than knowing where to shop for good prices and how to find a generic equivalent of a brand-name product. A smart consumer tries to live up to the following ancient dictum: *Know thyself.* To properly self-diagnose and self-treat, you need to know as much about yourself as possible.

Before taking any medications, read through the ingredients and identify whether or not you are allergic to any component in the product. Understandably, there's always a first time, so use remedies conservatively. If you are on a special diet, find out if that remedy works with your nutritional plans. And if you have existing medical problems, check to see if the OTC or natural remedy is safe for people with your condition, and if there is the possibility of an adverse drug interaction with other medications you may be taking.

Your Personal Medical Record

Just as your physician keeps your medical history in the office, you should consider keeping a personal medical history at home. This record includes information on all of your illnesses and operations (what you had, when you had it, how and when it was treated). In addition, write down what medications and supplements you take, and what allergies or sensitivities you may have.

If applicable, an account of pregnancies and births is very important. Keep a record of the vaccinations and booster shots you received, and the dates on which they were administered. Lifestyle issues are important, as well. For example, do you smoke cigarettes and/or drink alcohol? How much and for how long? Indicate any special nutritional needs you have. For instance, if you tend to have iron-deficiency anemia, be sure to write this on your record.

Family illnesses are an important part of a personal medical record. A list of the causes of death of close relatives may prove quite valuable to you at a later date. Finally, don't ignore your emotional life. Note any periods of depression or anxiety. If you have undergone major traumas—for example, divorce; death of a spouse, child, or parent; loss of a job—mark down when these events occurred and how you felt.

A personal medical record can be an extremely useful tool for the smart consumer. To make it easier for you to begin one, we have included a Personal Medical Record Form at the back of this book (see Appendix B, page 348). Photocopy this form and fill it in. Then be sure to give a copy to your pharmacist and to keep one in an accessible place in your home. Update this record at regular intervals.

CHILDREN AND REMEDIES

Certain precautions must be taken to prevent children from harming themselves by inappropriately taking OTCs and natural remedies. Keep all medicines out of children's reach, and use child-resistant caps on all products.

When treating a child, carefully follow the applicable instructions on the labels. Usually, specific doses will be suggested according to the child's age. Confirm or inquire about dosages through a pharmacist; *do not guess!* And always consult a physician when you are treating an infant.

Never give a child more than one medicine at the same time without checking with a doctor or a pharmacist. Furthermore, never give a child any OTC or natural remedy that is not recommended by a doctor or a pharmacist, or that is not specifically formulated for children (as confirmed on the label). And medicines should not be used for purposes other than those listed on the product label.

It is very important *not* to give aspirin or aspirin-containing products to a child or teenager who has a fever, who is recovering from the flu or the chickenpox, or who has flu symptoms—nausea, vomiting, elevated temperature. If the child has a viral infection and aspirin is given, Reye's syndrome could result. This is a serious illness that can affect many organs, including the brain and liver, and can even be fatal.

YOUR MEDICINE CHEST

It is helpful to have both OTC and natural remedies for common ailments in your medicine chest at home, ready for when they are needed. Remember to store your remedies out of the reach of children and in a dry place that is protected from light. Also, always check the expiration dates on all products, and discard those that have expired. Here's a sample list of what should be contained in a well-stocked medicine chest:

OTCs

- antacids
- antibiotic creams
- antidiarrheals
- antifungals
- antihistamines
- aspirin, acetaminophen, ibuprofen, or naproxen sodium
- calamine lotion
- cough/cold and flu medicine

- dimenhydrinate tablets (for motion sickness; allergic reactions)
- hydrocortisone cream
- hydrogen peroxide
- laxatives
- sunscreens

Natural Remedies

- aloe vera gel
- baking soda
- chamomile
- ginger
- echinacea
- peppermint tea
- psyllium (for fiber)
- witch hazel

In addition to OTCs and natural remedies, your medicine chest should also contain: adhesive bandages and tape; elastic bandages; gauze bandages; sterile nonstick dressings; cotton balls and rolls; antiseptic wipes; cold packs; insect repellent; disposable gloves; soaps; tongue depressors; tweezers; safety pins; scissors; and a thermometer.

PART TWO

An A-To-Z Guide To Common Conditions

It is important that you are aware of your many options when it comes to self-care. How much do you know about the products in the medicine aisle at your drug store? The commercials and magazine ads don't often address possible side effects. And have you considered vitamins and herbs as possible treatments for your self-managed conditions? When it comes to natural remedies, it's normal to wonder what is based on old wives' tales and what has been found to be scientifically reliable.

The truth is that there are many available and effective remedies to ease common conditions, but it's difficult to keep abreast of the latest in health care and to find the time to research all of your options. The writers of the *Pharmacist's Guide to Over-the-Counter and Natural Remedies* understand that you need clear, straightforward information. Simply turn to the condition that you want to know more about; the conditions are discussed alphabetically. You will find a definition of the condition and recommended over-the-counter and natural remedies. We have taken care to suggest only those remedies that have been researched and found to have a reasonable level of scientific validity.

Abscess

An abscess is a collection of pus in tissue, an organ, or a confined space in the body. Abscesses are usually the result of infections caused most frequently by bacteria, viruses, parasites, and fungi. They can form on almost any part of the body, both within the body and at the skin surface. The affected area of an abscess becomes swollen, inflamed, and tender. This is due to the accumulation of white blood cells that come to the site to combat the infection. Because the body is fighting pathogens, fever and chills often accompany this condition.

OTC REMEDIES

The products listed in the following table are analgesics—substances that reduce or relieve pain. These remedies also lower fever. If you have experienced side effects from any nonprescription pain relievers, do not take any of these products without consulting your doctor. Always read the label before using a product.

OTC Remedy	Dosage	Comments
Acetaminophen *Excedrin Aspirin-Free; Panadol; Tylenol*	325 mg regular strength; generally, 500 mg extra strength	Do not drink alcohol and use products containing acetaminophen. The combination can cause liver damage. Do not take this remedy with other analgesics. Some of these products, such as *Tylenol,* are available in junior, regular, and extra strength.

Aspirin (acetylsalicylic acid) *Ascriptin; Bayer; Bufferin; Ecotrin; Empirin; Excedrin Extra Strength*	325 mg regular strength; generally, 500 mg extra strength	If pregnant, consult your doctor before taking products containing aspirin. Do not take products containing aspirin during the last three months of pregnancy. Children and teens should not use products containing aspirin for colds, flus, or chickenpox. Do not take products containing aspirin if you have asthma, stomach problems, gastric ulcers, bleeding problems, or if you are allergic to aspirin.
Ibuprofen *Advil; Arthritis Foundation Ibuprofen; Motrin IB; Nuprin*	200 mg	If pregnant, consult your doctor before taking this remedy. Do not take products containing this ingredient during the last three months of pregnancy. Do not take this ingredient if you are allergic to aspirin. Do not take this ingredient with other analgesics. Consult your doctor before taking this remedy with prescription drugs.
Ketoprofen *Orudis*	12.5 mg	Same comments as Ibuprofen.
Naproxen sodium *Aleve*	220 mg	If pregnant, consult your doctor before taking this remedy. Do not take products containing this ingredient during the last three months of pregnancy. Do not take this ingredient with any other analgesics. Consult your doctor before taking this remedy with prescription drugs.

When used responsibly, acetaminophen, aspirin, ibuprofen, ketoprofen, and naproxen sodium are safe and effective. Look for single-ingredient products. If you have questions or concerns regarding the safety and effectiveness of any product, consult your doctor or pharmacist.

NATURAL REMEDIES

Abscesses should be treated both externally and internally. External treatment is necessary to release toxins and to encourage drainage. It should include soaking the affected area at least two times a day, for fifteen to thirty minutes. Water should be as hot as can be tolerated. It can be applied directly to the skin or by using a washcloth soaked in hot water. Hot baths are helpful. If desired, Epsom salts can be added to the water to increase the drawing out of the toxins. Also, ice packs can reduce painful swelling, if needed.

Internal treatment involves plenty of bed rest and the drinking of substantial amounts of water and other fluids. Drink green juices—for example, wheat grass juice, or 1 to 2 tablespoons of liquid chlorophyll (available at most health-food stores) added to water or juice—three times per day. It is also important to include cleansing foods in the diet, such as whole foods, vegetables, and fruits. Consuming sweets, and overeating in general, should be avoided. In addition, the nutrients listed in the following table should be part of your daily nutrition plan.

Natural Remedy	Dosage	Comments
Echinacea	*Dried extract:* 300 mg, 3 times daily, for 14 days *Fluid extract:* ½ tsp, 3 times daily for 14 days	Appears to lose its immune-boosting properties after a couple of weeks. It is most effective for short-term use.
Multivitamin/mineral*	See pages 14 to 20.	See pages 14 to 20.
Vitamin A*	25,000 IU daily, for 14 days only	Take with a meal. Can be toxic when taken in large amounts for a long period of time. Be sure to restrict this regimen to 14 days, unless a physician directs you otherwise.
Vitamin C*	1,000 mg, 3 times daily	Safe for long-term maintenance.
Vitamin E*	400 IU, daily	Take with a meal. Mixed tocopherols supplying 400 IU of d-alpha tocopherol are preferred. Can be used for long-term maintenance.

* It is important that the discussed nutrients be part of a basic vitamin/mineral regimen so that the total daily amount of each nutrient obtained from both a multivitamin/mineral and other supplements is approximately the dosage indicated above.

Occasionally, some abscesses are resistant to the methods of natural treatment outlined above. If this is the case, consult a physician. He or she may treat the abscess or boil by incising and draining the affected area, and may or may not prescribe an oral antibiotic.

Acid Indigestion

See Indigestion.

Acne

See also Skin Problems.

Acne is a common inflammatory skin disease. It is so prevalent among teenagers that it can almost be considered "normal." Acne affects about 80 percent of people between the ages of twelve and twenty-four. Superficial acne is characterized by blackheads (signifying partially-blocked pores) and/or whiteheads (indicating completely-blocked pores). In such cases, spontaneous remission is the rule. More serious forms of acne, often involving cystic growths, require consultation with a doctor.

Among factors that can be related to the onset and progression of acne are: hormones; oily skin; certain cosmetics; allergies; stress; excess junk food; chocolate; and oral contraceptives. Abrasive soaps should be avoided, and antibacterial soaps offer no benefit in treating this condition. Squeezing and pressing blemishes do more harm than good and can cause scarring.

OTC REMEDIES

There are a number of topical over-the-counter acne treatments. Generally, such products contain either benzoyl peroxide or salicylic acid. Always read the label before using a product.

OTC Remedy	Application	Comments
Benzoyl Peroxide		
Acne-Aid	As directed on label.	Mild reddening and drying of skin is common. If using both benzoyl peroxide and salicylic acid, allow 12 hours between the two treatments.
Clearasil zoyl Peroxide	As directed on label.	Same comments as *Acne-Ben-Aid.*
Exact zoyl Peroxide Acne Medication	As directed on label.	Same comments as *Acne-Ben-Aid.*
Oxy-10	As directed on label.	Same comments as *Acne-Aid.*
Salicylic Acid		
Stri-Dex Gel Acne Medication	As directed on label.	Pigment in the affected *Clear* area can temporarily change. Some peeling and stinging can occur. Do not use immediately before or after benzoyl peroxide treatment; allow 12 hours between these two acne treatments.
Stri-Dex Pads	As directed on label.	Same comments as *Stri-Dex Clear Gel Acne Medication.*

NATURAL REMEDIES

Acne appears on the skin when there is an imbalance within the body. It should therefore be treated both externally and internally. Care should be taken to avoid touching the affected area because of the risk of introducing bacteria. External treatment includes washing the affected area daily with a mild glycerin soap. To remove excess oil from the skin, soak a washcloth in very warm water and apply it to the affected area several times a day. Also, natural sunlight is one of the best treatments for acne.

Internal treatment includes avoiding high-fat, junk, and fast foods. Follow a cleansing diet that includes whole foods and fresh fruits and vegetables. The Five-A-Day Diet is a good eating plan (see page 21). Drinking green juices and six to eight glasses of water per day is highly recommended. In addition, the natural remedies listed in the table below will encourage the reduction of acne.

Natural Remedy	Dosage	Comments
Burdock root tea	3 to 6 cups, daily	A traditional blood-purifying tea; aids in the healing of skin disorders. Can interfere with iron absorption.
Chromium*	400 mcg, daily	Take with a meal. Involved in glucose metabolism and the synthesis of cholesterol, fats, and protein.
Flaxseed oil	*Liquid:* 1 tbsp, daily *Pill:* 1 capsule, 3 to 5 times daily	Supplies essential fatty acids; promotes healthy skin.
Multivitamin/ mineral*	See pages 14 to 20.	See pages 14 to 20.
Red clover tea	3 to 6 cups, daily	A traditional blood-purifying tea; aids in the healing of skin disorders.
Vitamin A*	25,000 IU daily, for 14 days only, then 10,000 IU daily.	Take with a meal. Can be toxic when taken in large amounts for a long

		period of time; be sure to restrict 25,000 IU regimen to 14 days, unless a physician directs you otherwise.
Vitamin B complex*	25 to 50 mg of all B vitamins, daily	Take with a meal. Safe for long-term maintenance.
Vitamin C*	1,000 mg, 3 times daily	Safe for long-term maintenance.
Vitamin E*	400 IU, daily	Take with a meal. Mixed tocopherols supplying 400 IU of d-alpha tocopherol are preferred. Can be used for long-term maintenance.
Zinc*	30 mg, daily	Take with a meal. Doses in excess of 100 mg can depress immune function.

* It is important that the discussed nutrients be part of a basic vitamin/mineral regimen so that the total daily amount of each nutrient obtained from both a multivitamin/mineral and other supplements is approximately the dosage indicated above.

Age Spots

Age spots are flat, brown spots—sometimes called "liver spots"—that can appear anywhere on the body. Several factors can play a role in the development of age spots, including: poor diet; lack of exercise; impaired liver function; and/or excessive exposure to the sun. Age spots indicate that waste products are accumulating and destroying brain and liver cells, as well as other cells, throughout the body. However, the spots themselves are considered harmless.

OTC REMEDIES

There are no recommended OTC products for lessening or removing the appearance of age spots. But for ways to possibly prevent age spots, see the following section on natural remedies.

NATURAL REMEDIES

In order to prevent age spots, limit your exposure to the sun. Also, avoid caffeine, processed and fried foods, tobacco, and sugar. Consume a balanced diet, and make sure that 50 percent of it is made up of the following raw fruits and vegetables, fresh grains, seeds, and nuts. In addition, the nutrition plan listed in the following table should help prevent the development of age spots.

Natural Remedy	Dosage	Comments
Grape-seed extract or **Pine bark extract** *Pycnogenol*	50 mg, daily	A potent antioxidant for the prevention of age spots. Grape-seed extract and pine bark extract are comparable substances.
Milk thistle extract	100 mg, 2 times daily	An excellent aid to maintaining healthy liver function. The best form is an extract bound to phosphatidylcholine. See product label.
Multivitamin/ mineral*	See pages 14 to 20.	See pages 14 to 20.
Vitamin C*	500 mg, 3 times daily	Safe for long-term maintenance.

* It is important that the discussed nutrients be part of a basic vitamin/mineral regimen so that the total daily amount of each nutrient obtained from both a multivitamin/mineral and other supplements is approximately the dosage indicated above.

Allergy

See also Food Allergy.

An allergy is actually an ineffective and inappropriate immune response to "innocent" chemical substances that are not usually harmful to the body. Asthma, eczema, and hay fever are frequent allergic responses. Common allergy-provoking items include: certain foods; certain types of material used in clothing; plants; pollen; metals; chemicals in soaps and cosmetics; food additives; dust; mold; animal hair or dander; and drugs.

No one knows what causes allergies or why certain substances are *allergens* (allergy-provoking substances) for one person and not for another. There is a hereditary factor to some people's allergies. In addition, some evidence suggests that emotional factors, such as stress or anger, play a role in the onset of allergies. Also, smoking can worsen allergies.

OTC REMEDIES

The products listed in the following table may be effective in relieving the symptoms of allergies. Those listed under acetaminophen and aspirin are analgesics—substances that relieve or reduce pain. If you have experienced side effects from any nonprescription pain relievers, do not take any analgesics without consulting your doctor. Always read the label before using a product.

OTC Remedy	Dosage	Comments
For General Allergy Relief		
Acetaminophen *Benadryl Allergy Sinus Headache; Children's Tylenol Cold Multi-SymptomChewable Tablets/Liquid; Children's Tylenol Cold Plus Cough Multi-Symptom Chewable Tablets/Liquid; Coricidin Tablets; Drixoral Cold & Flu Extended-Release Tablets; Sinarest Tablets; Sine-Off Caplets; Sinutab Caplets/ Tablets; Tylenol Cold Medicine Multi-Symptom Formula Tablets/ Caplets; Tylenol Severe Allergy Medication Caplets*	As directed on label.	Do not drink alcohol and use products containing acetamino-phen. The combination can cause liver damage. Do not take with other analgesics. Some acetaminophen products cause drowsiness; take necessary precautions and/or look for "no drowsiness" formulas. May cause dryness of mucous membranes; maintain fluid intake. Some of these products, such as *Sine-Off,* are available in regular and non-drowsiness formulas. Others, such as *Sinarest* and *Sinutab,* have maximum-/extra-strength formulas, in addition.
Actifed Allergy Daytime/Nighttime Caplets	As directed on label	Can cause drowsiness and dryness of mucous membranes. Take necessary precautions and maintain fluid intake.
Allerest Caplets	As directed on label.	Available in children's chewable tablets and 12-hour caplets. Can cause drowsiness and dryness of mucous membranes. Take necessary precautions and maintain fluid intake. May further irritate eyes, in which case use should be discontinued.

Aspirin (acetylsalicylic acid) *Alka-Seltzer Plus Sinus Medicine*	As directed on label.	If pregnant, consult your doctor before taking products containing aspirin. Do not take products containing aspirin during the last three months of pregnancy. Children and teens should not use products containing aspirin for colds, flus, or chickenpox. Do not take products containing aspirin if you have asthma, stomach problems, gastric ulcers, bleeding problems, or if you are allergic to aspirin. Can cause drowsiness and dryness of mucous membranes. Take necessary precautions and maintain fluid intake.
Benadryl Allergy Tablets/Kapseals/ Liquid	As directed on label.	Can cause drowsiness and dryness of the mucous . membranes Take necessary precautions and maintain fluid intake.
Chlor-Trimeton Allergy Tablets	As directed on label.	Available in 4-, 8-, and 12-hour formulas. Can cause drowsiness and dryness of the mucous membranes. Take necessary precautions and maintain fluid intake.
Contac 12-Hour Timed Release Capsules	As directed on label.	Can cause drowsiness and dryness of the mucous membranes. Take necessary precautions and maintain fluid intake.
Dimetapp Tablets/Liqui-gels/ Elixir	As directed on label.	Can cause drowsiness and dryness of the mucous membranes. Take necessary precautions and maintain fluid intake.

Drixoral Cold & Allergy Sustained-Action Tablets	As directed on label.	Can cause drowsiness and dryness of the mucous membranes. Take necessary precautions and maintain fluid intake.
Efidac 24	As directed on label.	Can cause drowsiness and dryness of mucous membranes. Take necessary precautions and maintain fluid intake.
PediaCare Cold/Allergy Chewable Tablets	As directed on label.	Can cause drowsiness and dryness of mucous membranes. Take necessary precautions and maintain fluid intake.
PediaCare Cough-Cold Liquid/Chewable Tablets	As directed on label.	Can cause drowsiness and dryness of mucous membranes. Take necessary precautions and maintain fluid intake.
Sudafed Caplets/ Tablets/Liquid	As directed on label.	Available in regular strength (30 mg), adult strength (60 mg), children's, 12-hour, and *Plus* formulas. Some formulas can cause drowsiness and dryness of the mucous membranes. Take necessary precautions and maintain fluid intake.
Tavist-1 Tablets	As directed on label.	Can cause drowsiness and dryness of mucous membranes. Take necessary precautions and maintain fluid intake.
Tavist-D Tablets	As directed on label.	Can cause drowsiness and dryness of mucous membranes. Take necessary precautions and maintain fluid intake.
Triaminic Syrup/Tablets	As directed on label.	Available in regular syrup, cold tablets, and allergy tablets. Can cause drowsiness and dryness of mucous membranes. Take necessary precautions and maintain fluid intake.

Triaminic-12 Tablets	As directed on label.	Can cause drowsiness and dryness of the mucous membranes. Take necessary precautions and maintain fluid intake.

For Relief From Nasal Congestion

Actifed	As directed on label.	Available in several formulas. Combination decongestant and antihistamine. Can cause drowsiness and dryness of the mucous membranes. Take necessary precautions and maintain fluid intake.
Afrin Nasal Spray/ Spray Pump/ Sinus Nasal Spray	As directed on label.	Can cause nasal irritation and dryness in some individuals.
Cheracol Nasal Spray Pump	As directed on label.	Can cause nasal irritation and dryness in some individuals.
Chlor-Trimeton Allergy/ Decongestant Tablets	As directed on label.	Available in 4- and 12-hour formulas. Can cause drowsiness and dryness of the mucous membranes. Take necessary precautions and maintain fluid intake.
4-Way Nasal Spray	As directed on label.	Available in *Fast-Acting* and *Long-Lasting* formulas. Can cause nasal irritation and dryness in some individuals.
Neo-Synephrine Drops/Sprays	As directed on label.	Available in pediatric, regular, adult, 12-hour, and long-acting formulas. Can cause headache and nasal irritation and dryness in some individuals.
PediaCare Infants' Oral Decongestant Drops	As directed on label.	No common side effects. Consult a doctor if a reaction occurs, such as vomiting, difficulty breathing, insomnia, or agitation.

Vicks Sinex	As directed on label.	Can cause headache and nasal irritation and dryness in some individuals.
Vicks Sinex 12-Hour Formula Decongestant Nasal Spray	As directed on label.	Can cause nasal irritation and dryness in some individuals.

If you are interested in a product containing acetaminophen or aspirin, know that when used responsibly, these substances are safe and effective. Look for single-ingredient products. If you have questions or concerns regarding the safety and effectiveness of any product, consult your doctor or pharmacist.

While these OTC remedies may be effective, the first line of defense and most preferable treatment for allergies should be to identify specific allergens and remove them from the environment. In many cases, medication is not needed.

NATURAL REMEDIES

Below are listed several nutrients and natural substances that may help to relieve allergy symptoms. For more information, consult a nutritionist who specializes in allergies.

Natural Remedy	Dosage	Comments
Bioflavonoids	1,000 mg, daily	Nutrients that serve many functions, some of which are the reduction of pain, maintenance of capillary health, and antibacterial action. Quercetin is a specific bioflavonoid that may be effective against asthma symptoms.

Grape-seed extract or **Pine bark extract** *Pycnogenol*	25 mg, daily	Potent antioxidant. Grape-seed extract and pine bark extract are comparable substances.
Multivitamin/ mineral*	See pages 14 to 20.	See pages 14 to 20.
Nasixx	4 to 8 tablets, 3 times daily	A traditional Chinese herbal formula found in drug and health-food stores.
Pantothenic acid*	500 mg, daily	Also known as vitamin B_5 and an "anti-stress" vitamin. Deficiency has been found to adversely affect the immune system.
Vitamin B_6*	50 mg, 2 times daily	Check your multivitamin/ mineral label and add extra vitamin B_6 so that total daily dosage is approximately 100 mg.
Vitamin C*	1,000 mg, 3 times daily	Safe for long-term maintenance.
Vitamin E*	400 IU, daily	Take with a meal. Mixed tocopherols supplying 400 IU of d-alpha tocopherol are preferred. Safe for long-term maintenance.

* It is important that the discussed nutrients be part of a basic vitamin/mineral regimen so that the total daily amount of each nutrient obtained from both a multivitamin/mineral and other supplements is approximately the dosage indicated above.

Alopecia

See Hair and Scalp Problems.

Anemia

Anemia is characterized by a decrease in the number of red blood cells (RBCs) or in hemoglobin content in the blood. It is due to blood loss, impaired production of RBCs, or a combination of these factors. Early signs include loss of appetite, constipation, irritability, and headaches. Common symptoms are weakness, fatigue, dizziness, pallor, drowsiness, and the cessation of menstruation. Millions of Americans are anemic. About 50 percent of those with this condition are children; approximately 20 percent are women.

One of the factors that contributes to the development of anemia is iron deficiency. Risk of iron deficiency is high during a child's years of growth, when a girl reaches puberty and begins menstruation, and during pregnancy. However, bleeding—not poor diet or the above discussed stages of life—is the most frequent cause of iron deficiency.

Anemia is not really a condition in itself. It is part of a complex of signs and symptoms. Even a mild case of anemia needs thorough investigation by a doctor because the presence of anemia indicates the existence of an underlying disorder. Sophisticated laboratory work is necessary to uncover the origin and significance of the anemia. Hormonal disorders, infection, dietary deficiency, and serious physical illness (for example, thyroid, diverticular, liver, and bone marrow diseases) may be involved.

OTC REMEDIES

If, upon the advice of your physician, you will be supplementing with iron, you can find this mineral in a variety of multivitamins/minerals and in separate supplements. Current opinion in the pharmaceutical field designates supplements that contain iron as over-the-counter remedies. The supplements listed in the following chart are suggested multivitamins plus iron. There are a number of children's supplements that contain iron, as well. However, due to the importance of contacting a physician before supplementing children's diets with iron, we have chosen not to list any products here.

OTC Remedy	Dosage	Comments
Centrum Multivitamin-Multimineral Formula	As directed on label.	Take with a meal. Available in *Jr.* and *Silver* (for adults 50 years of age and older) formulas, as well.
Theragran M Multivitamin with Minerals Tablets	As directed on label.	Take with a meal.

Use caution when supplementing with iron, and do so only under a doctor's careful supervision. Excess iron is the most frequent form of poisoning today. You must seek a doctor's direction and have blood tests done to evaluate your iron levels before deciding on a supplement regimen. If a female takes a multivitamin/mineral plus iron, the results are usually safe. Children and men are at greater risk for iron poisoning. In fact, *iron poisoning is now the number-one cause of poisoning among children.*

NATURAL REMEDIES

For many iron-deficient anemics, the bottom line is that although it takes more time and thought, getting the proper amount of iron and other nutrients through diet may be the best choice. An experienced nutritionist can help you create a healthy eating plan. Include the following iron-rich foods in your diet: broccoli; blackstrap molasses; egg yolks; kelp; leafy green vegetables; peas; parsley; prunes; raisins; rice bran; turnip greens; and whole grains, but not bran. Eating fish at the same time as vegetables increases iron absorption. Also, foods that are high in vitamin C, such as berries, citrus fruits, and green vegetables, aid in iron absorption. The richest sources of iron are liver and other organ meats, lean beef, dried fruits, and lima beans.

Anxiety

See Mood Disorders.

Appetite Disturbances

An appetite disturbance involves a change in normal food cravings and eating patterns. A number of factors can cause a disturbance in appetite, including:

depression; stress and emotional trauma; an unpleasant environment; use and misuse of alcohol and drugs (both licit and illicit); smoking; certain medical conditions; and certain medications. After a period of disturbed appetite, secondary problems may set in. For example, an ordinary meal may look like a very large amount of food to a person who has been eating too little. As a result, just the sight of the meal may be overwhelming and cause a loss of appetite. Also, keep in mind that an appetite disturbance may be a sign of a serious psychological problem such as anorexia or bulimia, which are severe eating disorders that require medical attention.

OTC TREATMENTS

There are no recommended OTC products that trigger appetite or reduce the anxiety of appetite disturbance. However, see below for helpful natural remedies.

NATURAL REMEDIES

Appetite disturbances must be handled individually; there is no standard method to restore a normal desire for food in a person. Such factors as personal taste in food, the appearance of the meal, and the environment in which the meal is served are crucial and must be tailored to the satisfaction of the individual. But for poor appetite, some options include not drinking liquids before or during meals, and performing moderate exercise daily.

Eat small portions of raw fruits and vegetables as often as possible. Avoid "quick fixes" with candy, donuts, and other junk foods. Also, supplementing once daily with 30 milligrams of zinc, taken with food, may help to regain appetite and taste. This level of zinc should not be taken daily for long periods of time, as it can deplete the body of copper.

Arthritis

Inflammation and/or pain in the joints of the hips, knees, toes, neck, back, shoulders, elbows, wrists, and fingers are characteristic of arthritis. For those who suffer from this condition, swelling and stiffness in the joints are common. Deformity can occur with severe, prolonged arthritis. Pain may be sudden and sharp, or it may be gradual and dull. Poor nutrition, bacterial infection, and physical and emotional stress can play a role in the onset and severity of arthritis.

This condition appears in a number of different forms; osteoarthritis, rheumatoid arthritis, and juvenile rheumatoid arthritis are the most common. Osteoarthritis tends to affect a specific joint or joints. About 16 million Americans have osteoarthritis, also known as degenerative joint disease. Osteoarthritis seems to run in families, and afflicts three times as many women as men. Rheumatoid arthritis affects the entire body. Over 2 million Americans suffer from rheumatoid arthritis, which afflicts twice as many women as men. And about 70,000 Americans under the age of eighteen suffer from juvenile rheumatoid arthritis; six times as many girls as boys have this condition. Gout, ankylosing spondylitis, and systemic lupus erythematosus are other prevalent types of arthritis, and are also more common in women.

OTC REMEDIES

The products listed in the following table may relieve the pain, soreness, and stiffness associated with arthritis. Those listed in the first section of the table are analgesics—substances that relieve or reduce pain. If you have experienced side effects from any nonprescription pain relievers, do not take any of these remedies without consulting your doctor. Always read the label before using a product.

OTC Remedy	Dosage/Application	Comments
Oral Pain-Relieving Medications		
Acetaminophen *Excedrin Aspirin-Free; Panadol; Tylenol*	325 mg regular strength; generally, 500 mg extra strength	Do not drink alcohol and use products containing acetaminophen. The combination can cause liver damage. Do not take with other analgesics. Some products, such as *Tylenol*, are available in junior, regular, and extra strength.
Aspirin (acetylsalicylic acid) *Ascriptin;Bayer; Bufferin;Ecotrin; Empirin; Excedrin Extra Strength*	325 mg regular strength; generally, 500 mg extra strength	If pregnant, consult your doctor before taking products containing aspirin. Do not take products containing aspirin during the last three months of pregnancy. Children and teens should not use products containing aspirin for colds, flus, or chickenpox. Do not take products containing aspirin if you have asthma,

		stomach problems; gastric ulcers, bleeding problems, or if you are allergic to aspirin.
Ibuprofen *Advil; Arthritis Foundation Ibuprofen; Motrin IB; Nuprin*	200 mg	If pregnant, consult your doctor before taking this remedy. Do not take products containing this ingredient during the last three months of pregnancy. Do not take this ingredient if you are allergic to aspirin. Do not take this ingredient with any other analgesics. Consult your doctor before taking this remedy with prescription drugs.
Ketoprofen *Orudis KT*	12.5 mg	Same comments as Ibuprofen.
Naproxen sodium *Aleve*	220 mg	If pregnant, consult your doctor before taking this remedy. Do not take products containing this ingredient during the last three months of pregnancy. Do not take this ingredient with any other analgesics. Consult your doctor before taking this remedy with prescription drugs.

Topical Products

Bengay Pain-Relieving Ointment/Cream	As directed on label.	Available in the original ointment and in a greaseless cream. Do not apply to broken or irritated skin.
Capsaicin *Capzasin-P Topical Analgesic Cream*	As directed on label.	Do not apply to broken or irritated skin.

When used responsibly, acetaminophen, aspirin, ibuprofen, ketoprofen, and naproxen sodium are safe and effective. Look for single-ingredient products. If you have questions or concerns regarding the safety and effectiveness of any product, consult your doctor or pharmacist.

NATURAL REMEDIES

Making changes in the diet can be an effective way to treat or eliminate the joint inflammation that accompanies both osteoarthritis and rheumatoid arthritis. To reduce symptoms, eliminate "nightshade" plants from the diet for a period of three months. These include: tomatoes, potatoes, peppers, eggplant, and tobacco. In addition, following a diet that eliminates all regularly-eaten foods for a period of three weeks may help you identify any food substances that might be worsening your condition. (See Food Allergy, page 188.) For osteoarthritis, calcium pantothenate has been found helpful. It is obtainable through whole grains and legumes, or through supplementation (see the following chart). Finally, the nutrient supplements listed below are a natural way to boost well-being and to reduce the symptoms of arthritis.

Natural Remedy	Dosage	Comments
For Osteoarthritis and Rheumatoid Arthritis		
EPA Fish Oil	1,000 mg, daily	Take with food.
Hydrolyzed gelatin *Knox NutraJoint; Arthred G*	1 scoop, daily, mixed in favorite beverage	Natural hydrolyzed collagen (gelatin) helps to build and maintain healthy joint components. It requires daily use for two months to achieve

		optimal effect.
Multivitamin/ mineral*	See pages 14 to 20.	See pages 14 to 20.
Rheumixx	4 tablets, 3 times daily	A traditional Chinese herbal formula found in most drug stores.
Vitamin C*	1,000 mg, 3 times daily	Safe for long-term maintenance.
Vitamin E*	400 IU, daily	Take with a meal. Mixed tocopherols supplying 400 IU of d-alpha tocopherol are preferred. Safe for long-term maintenance.
For Osteoarthritis Only		
Calcium pantothenate	100 mg, daily	Keep in mind that you can receive this nutrient through diet, instead of supplements. Under doctor's supervision, dosage may go as high as 2,000 mg daily.
Glucosamine	500 to 1,000 mg, 3 times daily	This ingredient may be combined with chondroitin— a constituent of cartilage—as in brands such as *Osteo-Bi-Flex*. Must be taken for a minimum of two months in order to get full effects.

* It is important that the discussed nutrients be part of a basic vitamin/mineral regimen so that the total daily amount of each nutrient obtained from both a multivitamin/mineral and other supplements is approximately the dosage indicated above.

Asthma

Asthma is a lung condition characterized by an obstruction of the breathing airways. Inflammation of the airways is usually present during an attack, as well as chronically in the asthmatic individual, and the airways have an increased responsiveness to a variety of stimuli. An asthma attack is generally triggered by a number of factors in combination. Among them are spasms of the smooth muscles in the airways; swelling of the mucosae; and increased secretion of mucus. Chronic asthma is truly an inflammatory disease.

Allergens (allergy-provoking substances) of any kind can induce an asthma attack. The body produces *histamine* in response to the allergens, which causes the muscle spasms and increased mucus production. Common symptoms of asthma include difficulty breathing, tightness in the chest, coughing, and wheezing. Asthma can be reversed by treatment, and sometimes asthma reverses itself spontaneously. Regardless, it is a serious condition requiring a doctor's attention.

There are about 10 million Americans who suffer from asthma. From 1970 to 1987, hospitalization rates for this condition tripled in the United States. In the 1980s, the number of asthmatics grew by 29 percent. African-Americans were over twice as likely to need hospitalization for this condition as Caucasian Americans. Also in that decade, asthma death rates in the United States tripled. And the situation has only worsened. The number of individuals afflicted with this condition continues to rise, partly due to increases in pollution.

OTC REMEDIES

Luckily, there are OTC products that can provide symptomatic relief from asthma, including those listed in the following table.

OTC Remedy	Dosage	Comments
Bronkaid Caplets/Mist	As directed on label.	Dilates the bronchial tubes; reduces congestion and the release of histamine. Do not take with drugs containing ephedrine, pseudoephedrine, or epinephrine. Consult with your doctor before using, and before combining this treatment with other medications. Common side effects include nervousness, trembling, and dryness in the throat or mouth. More severe reactions, such as headache, vomiting, palpitations, dizziness, sleep problems, difficulty breathing, and rashes are not common, but occur in some individuals. Consult a doctor if you experience a reaction.
Primatene Dual-Action Formula Tablets	As directed on label.	Contains ephedrine; dilates the bronchial tubes; reduces congestion and the release of histamine. Do not take with MAO inhibitors; if allergic to ephedrine, or similar drugs, bronchodilators, or barbituates; or if you have a stomach ulcer. Consult with your doctor before using and before combining this treatment with other medications. Common side effects include such symptoms as headache, nervousness, irritability, insomnia, vomiting, dizziness, and

		heartburn. More severe reactions, such as rashes, diarrhea, confusion, pain, fever, and oral sores are not common but have been known to occur. Consult a physician if you experience a reaction.
Primatene Mist/Tablets	As directed on label.	Same comments as *Bronkaid Caplets/Mist.*

Do not self-diagnose asthma and be careful not to overuse any of the above OTC products. Eventual resistance to many products is common. If you have questions or concerns regarding the safety and effectiveness of any product, consult your doctor or pharmacist. Valid concerns have been expressed by authorities in the consumer-health field regarding the safety and effectiveness of products that contain certain chemicals. The following warning has been issued:

• Do not use products that contain only guaifenesin and theophylline.

NATURAL REMEDIES

Avoid foods containing sulfites and other food additives and preservatives, as these substances can aggravate asthma. Eat plenty of fresh fruits and vegetables, especially onions, nuts and seeds, oatmeal, brown rice, and whole grains. Furthermore, eliminate sugar from your diet. Below are listed a number of nutrient supplements that also may help to alleviate asthma.

Natural Remedy	Dosage	Comments
Citrus bioflavonoids	1,000 mg, daily	Nutrients that serve many functions, some of which are pain reduction, maintenance of capillary health, and antibacterial action. Make sure that the combination contains quercetin, a bioflavonoid that has been found to be effective against asthma symptoms.
Grape-seed extract or **Pine bark extract** *Pycnogenol*	25 mg, 2 times daily	Potent antioxidant. Grape-seed extract or pine bark extract are comparable substances.
Magnesium*	400 mg, daily	Be sure your supplement regimen contains enough magnesium to reach this total daily dosage.
Multivitamin/ mineral*	See pages 14 to 20.	See pages 14 to 20.
Vitamin B$_{12}$ *	1,000 mcg, daily	Injections of this vitamin may also be helpful, especially to older individuals who may not be able to absorb oral vitamin B$_{12}$. For more information, consult your physician.
Vitamin C*	1,000 mg, 3 times daily	Safe for long-term maintenance.

* It is important that the discussed nutrients be part of a basic vitamin/mineral regimen so that the total daily amount of each nutrient obtained from both a multivitamin/mineral and other supplements is approximately the dosage indicated above.

Athlete's Foot

Athlete's foot is a fungal infection that thrives in warm, dark, damp environments. This condition, also known as *tinea pedis,* is quite common, especially during warm weather. It can spread rapidly in gyms, health clubs, and swimming-pool locker rooms. Common symptoms affecting the feet include inflammation, itching, a burning sensation, scaling of the skin, and sometimes blisters.

If an individual is taking antibiotics for a different condition, this may allow the fungal infection to spread more rapidly. Other drugs and radiation therapy may have a similar effect. (All of these forms of treatment destroy beneficial bacteria in addition to the harmful ones.) Prevention is paramount. The feet should be protected at all times from direct contact with the floor in places where exposure to the fungus that causes this condition is likely.

OTC REMEDIES

The following chart lists several topical OTC products that help combat athlete's foot. Always read the label before using a product.

OTC Remedy	Application	Comments
Aftate Antifungal Spray Powder for Athlete's Foot	As directed on label.	No common side effects. Increased irritation due to use of this product is infrequent.
Desenex Antifungal Powder/ Spray Powder/ Cream/Ointment/ Spray Liquid	As directed on label.	Also available in *Prescription Strength.* No common side effects. Increased irritation due to use of this product is infrequent.

| Lotrimin Antifungal Cream/Solution/ Lotion | As directed on label. | No common side effects. Increased irritation due to use of this product is infrequent. |
| Tinactin Antifungal Cream/Solution/ Liquid Aerosol/ Powder Aerosol/ Deodorant Powder Aerosol | As directed on label. | No common side effects. Increased irritation, itching, redness, etc., due to use of this product is infrequent. |

NATURAL REMEDIES

Hygiene and caution will prevent and resolve this condition most of the time. Purchase footwear to protect your feet from contact with fungi at the gym or health club. Bathe or shower immediately after exercise and dry the affected area thoroughly. It is important to maintain a healthy immune system, as this will decrease the incidence of chronic conditions. Follow the Five-A-Day Diet (see page 21) for good nutrition, get adequate rest, and exercise regularly. Follow a multivitamin/mineral regimen that includes the dosages of vitamins A, C, E, and the mineral zinc that are recommended in the table below.

Natural Remedy	Dosage	Comments
Vitamin A*	10,000 IU, daily	Take with a meal. A good multivitamin/mineral will contain this amount. Toxicity can result from higher doses taken for long periods of time.
Vitamin C*	500 mg, 3 times daily	Safe for long-term maintenance.

Vitamin E*	400 IU, daily	Take with a meal. Mixed tocopherols supplying 400 IU of d-alpha tocopherol are preferred. Can be used for long-term maintenance.
Zinc*	30 mg, daily	Take with a meal. Doses in excess of 100 mg can depress immune function.

* It is important that the discussed nutrients be part of a basic vitamin/mineral regimen so that the total daily amount of each nutrient obtained from both a multivitamin/mineral and other supplements is approximately the dosage indicated above.

Back Pain

Approximately 80 percent of Americans will experience back pain at some point in life. Back pain can be caused by a number of factors, some of which are: poor posture; poor muscle conditioning; overuse and sprains of muscles; strains of ligaments; improper footwear; a mattress that is too soft; incorrect lifting of heavy items; obesity; and pregnancy. Certain medical conditions can also cause back pain: arthritis; bone disease; slipped or ruptured discs; pelvic inflammatory disease; kidney or bladder problems; and curvature of the spine. In some cases, stress and/or psychological factors may play a role.

Back pain is often felt in the lower back, and is frequently accompanied by another condition called *sciatica*—a disorder involving pain radiating down one or both buttocks, or one or both legs, along the sciatic nerve. Acute pain following muscle strain is the most common form of back pain and usually clears up with relaxation of the muscle spasm, bed rest, and a pain-relieving drug. Chronic pain requires alleviating the cause of the back pain (for example, losing excess weight). An analgesic may help with the pain. If back pain persists for three or more days, or if the pain spreads into the legs, see a doctor.

OTC REMEDIES

The products listed in the first part of the following table are analgesics—substances that relieve or reduce pain. If you have experienced side effects from any nonprescription pain relievers, do not take any of these remedies without consulting your doctor. The second part of the table recommends topical products. Always read the label before using a product.

OTC Remedy	Dosage/Application	Comments
Oral Pain-Relieving Medications		
Acetaminophen *Excedrin Aspirin-Free; Panadol; Tylenol*	325 mg regular strength; generally, 500 mg extra strength	Do not drink alcohol and use products containing acetaminophen. The combination can cause liver damage. Do not take with other analgesics. Some of these products, such as *Tylenol,* are available in junior, regular, and extra strength.
Aspirin (acetylsalicylic acid) *Ascriptin; Bayer; Bufferin; Ecotrin; Empirin; Excedrin Extra Strength*	325 mg regular strength; generally, 500 mg extra strength	If pregnant, consult your doctor before taking products containing aspirin. Do not take products containing containing aspirin during the last three months of pregnancy. Children and teens should not use products containing aspirin for colds, flus, or chickenpox.

		Do not take products containing aspirin if you have asthma, stomach problems, gastric ulcers, bleeding problems, or if you are allergic to aspirin.
Ibuprofen *Advil; Arthritis Foundation Ibuprofen; Motrin IB; Nuprin*	200 mg	If pregnant, consult your doctor before taking this remedy. Do not take products containing this ingredient during the last three months of pregnancy. Do not take this ingredient if you are allergic to aspirin. Do not take this ingredient with any other analgesics. Consult your doctor before taking this remedy with prescription drugs.
Ketoprofen *Orudis KT*	12.5 mg	Same comments as Ibuprofen.
Magnesium salicylate *Doan's Regular Strength*	377 mg regular strength; 580 mg extra strength	Do not take with tetracyclines; consult with a doctor before combining with other medications. Common side effects include indigestion and ringing in the ears. If nausea, vomiting, or pain in the abdomen occur, seek immediate medical attention. More serious side effects, such as breathing problems, rashes, fever, very dark stools, and headache, are not common, but if they occur, a doctor's treatment is necessary.
Naproxen sodium *Aleve*	220 mg	If pregnant, consult your doctor before taking this remedy. Do not take products containing this ingredient during the last three months of pregnancy.

		Do not take this ingredient with any other analgesics. Consult your doctor before taking this remedy with prescription drugs.
Topical Products		
Bengay Pain-Relieving Ointment/Cream	As directed on label.	Available in original ointment and a greaseless cream. Do not apply to broken or irritated skin.
Capsaicin Capzasin-P Topical Analgesic Creme	As directed on label.	Do not apply to broken or irritated skin.

When used responsibly, acetaminophen, aspirin, ibuprofen, ketoprofen, magnesium salicylate, and naproxen sodium are safe and effective. Look for single-ingredient products. If you have questions or concerns regarding the safety and effectiveness of any product, consult your doctor or pharmacist.

NATURAL REMEDIES

An alternative to taking medication is to see a doctor or allied health practitioner, such as a physical therapist, about a supervised exercise program. On the road to recovery, and for preventing future incidences, you will need to strengthen your stomach muscles, side muscles, and back muscles. For proper guidance on stretching and strengthening the appropriate muscles, you can also consult an instructor such a chiropractor or a sports massage therapist. While your back is mending, you may find it more comfortable sleeping on your back with a pillow under your knees.

Bad Breath

This condition, also called *halitosis*, is characterized by an unpleasant odor to the breath. The odor may be produced by foods or drinks; tooth decay; dental disease; food particles caught between the teeth; bacteria in the mouth; or by a more serious underlying illness. A person may be unaware of having bad breath and, consequently, unaware of its impact on co-workers, family, and friends.

OTC REMEDIES

There are a number of products on the market that aim to freshen breath and cleanse the oral environment. Some recommended products include *Cepacol Mouthwash and Gargle* and *Listerine Antiseptic*. Mouthwashes and gargles often contain alcohol, but there are products that do not, such as *Listermint Alcohol-Free Mouthwash*.

NATURAL REMEDIES

Bad breath can be relieved by brushing the teeth and the tongue after every meal, and by using dental floss, wooden toothpicks, and mouthwash. Also, making a few changes to the diet can help eliminate chronic bad breath. Drink plenty of water—48 to 64 ounces per day. Increase the amount of fiber in the diet by eating plenty of fresh fruits and vegetables. Gargle with and drink green juices, such as wheat grass juice or liquid chlorophyll (1 to 2 tablespoons added to water or juice, taken a few times daily). These are available at most health-food stores. For occasional bad breath, chewing parsley can freshen the mouth.

Baldness

See Hair and Scalp Problems.

Bee Stings

Stinging insects are indigenous to every part of the country. Honeybees, bumblebees, yellow jackets, hornets, and wasps are dreaded for their stings, while spiders and ants commonly sting, as well. Symptoms resulting from a bee sting can include inflammation of the affected area, hoarseness, difficulty swallowing or breathing, swelling, and weakness. After a sting, the stinger should be "teased" out of the body—a better technique than scraping or pulling the stinger out. Ice will reduce swelling and pain.

Although it takes more than 1,000 bee stings to kill the average adult, a hypersensitive person can die from an *anaphylactic shock* reaction to a single bee sting. In such a reaction, the body responds by releasing histamine and other inflammatory substances. The inflammation can severely restrict breathing and may dilate blood vessels, causing blood pressure to drop dangerously low. The heart may malfunction as well, beating erratically and failing to sufficiently pump blood. Shock and unconsciousness often result.

There are three to four times more deaths in the United States from bee stings each year than from snakebites. In urban areas, up to 40 percent of the population may be stung by bees each year. People with known hypersensitivity to bee stings should carry an emergency kit (a doctor can prescribe one) with an antihistamine and a prefilled syringe containing aqueous epinephrine (that is, epinephrine in water), especially in areas where bees are common. Yet fortunately, for many of us, bee stings are just painful nuisances that can be self-treated.

OTC REMEDIES

The topical treatments listed in the following table are manufactured to relieve pain and itching. Always read the label before using a product.

OTC Remedy	Application	Comments
Americaine Topical Anesthetic Spray/First Aid Ointment	As directed on label.	Temporarily blocks the pain messages sent from the skin to the brain. No common side effects. Further skin irritation (possibly including hives) is unusual.
Benadryl Itch Relief Cream/ Spray/Gel	As directed on label.	Also available in maximum strength and children's formulas.
BiCozene Creme	As directed on label.	Topical anti-infective. No common side effects. Further skin irritation is unusual.
Caladryl Lotion	As directed on label.	Also available in *Cream for Kids* formula.

Caldecort Anti-Itch Cream/Spray	As directed on label	Also available in *Light Cream*. Reduces inflammation. No common side effects. Further skin irritation is unusual. Do not use if you are allergic to cortisone products.
Cortaid Cream/ Ointment/Spray	As directed on label.	The regular- and maximum-strength formulas are available in cream and ointment forms, while the maximum-strength formula is also available in spray form. Reduces inflammation. No common side effects. Further skin irritation is unusual. Do not use if you are allergic to cortisone products.
Cortizone for Kids	As directed on label.	Reduces inflammation. No common side effects. Further skin irritations occur only infrequently. Do not use if you are allergic to cortisone products.
Cortizone-5 Creme/Ointment	As directed on label.	Same comments as *Cortizone for Kids*.
Cortizone-10 Creme/Ointment	As directed on label.	Same comments as *Cortizone for Kids*.

If you have questions or concerns regarding the safety and effectiveness of any product, consult your doctor or pharmacist.

NATURAL REMEDIES

After removing the stinger, treat the affected area with a paste made from a little cool water added to any one of the following: baking soda; crushed aspirin;

crushed papaya-enzyme (papain) tablet; or meat tenderizer, which contains papain. Any of these pastes will help reduce the pain associated with bee stings and other insect bites.

Bladder Infection

See Cystitis.

Boils

See also Abscess.

This condition consists of what are known as *furuncles*—acute, tender, inflamed, round, pus-filled areas of skin, usually caused by infection with staphylococcus bacteria. Poor hygiene, stress, poor nutrition, illness, an infected wound, some drugs, and lowered immune function can all result in boils. This condition frequently occurs on the neck, breasts, face, scalp, underarms, and buttocks. Boils are most painful when they occur on the nose, ears, and fingers.

Boils are common in healthy, young individuals and may be recurrent. Common symptoms include itching, localized swelling, and pain. In general, boils appear suddenly and become red and filled with pus within a day. If boils occur near lymph glands, there may be swelling of those glands as well. Usually, a boil will heal in two to four weeks. Severe boils may require treatment by a doctor.

OTC TREATMENTS

The products listed in the following chart are analgesics—substances that relieve or reduce pain. They also combat fever. If you have experienced side effects from any nonprescription pain relievers, do not take any of these remedies without consulting your doctor. Always read the label before using a product.

OTC Remedy	Dosage	Comments
Acetaminophen *Excedrin Aspirin-Free; Panadol; Tylenol*	325 mg regular strength, generally, 500 mg extra strength	Do not drink alcohol and use products containing acetaminophen. The combination can cause liver damage. Do not take with other analgesics. Some of these products, such as *Tylenol,* are available in regular, junior, and extra strength.
Aspirin (acetylsalicylic acid) *Ascriptin; Bayer; Bufferin; Ecotrin; Empirin; Excedrin Extra Strength*	325 mg regular strength; generally, 500 mg extra strength	If pregnant, consult your doctor before taking products containing aspirin. Do not take products containing aspirin during the last three months of pregnancy. Children and teens should not use products containing aspirin for colds, flus, or chickenpox. Do not take products containing aspirin if you have asthma, stomach problems, gastric ulcers, bleeding problems, or if you are allergic to aspirin.

Ibuprofen *Advil; Arthritis Foundation Ibuprofen; Motrin IB; Nuprin*	200 mg	If pregnant, consult your doctor before taking this remedy. Do not take products containing this ingredient during the last three months of pregnancy. Do not take this ingredient if you are allergic to aspirin. Do not take this ingredient with any other analgesics. Consult your doctor before taking this remedy with prescription drugs.
Ketoprofen *Orudis KT*	12.5 mg	Same comments as Ibuprofen.
Naproxen sodium *Aleve*	220 mg	If pregnant, consult your doctor before taking this remedy. Do not take products containing this ingredient during the last three months of pregnancy. Do not take this ingredient with any other analgesics. Consult your doctor before taking this remedy with prescription drugs.

When used responsibly, acetaminophen, aspirin, ibuprofen, ketoprofen, and naproxen sodium are safe and effective. Look for single-ingredient products. If you have questions or concerns regarding the safety and effectiveness of any product, consult your doctor or pharmacist.

NATURAL REMEDIES

Boils should be treated both externally and internally. External treatment is necessary to release toxins and to encourage drainage. It should include soaking the affected area in water at least two times a day, for fifteen to thirty minutes. Water should be as hot as can be tolerated. You can apply it directly to the skin or use a washcloth soaked in hot water. If desired, Epsom salts can be added to the water to increase the drawing out of the toxins.

Internal treatment involves drinking substantial amounts of water and other fluids. Drink green juices, such as wheat grass juice and liquid chlorophyll (1 to 2 tablespoons added to water or juice, three times a day), which are available at most health-food stores. It is also important to include cleansing foods in the diet, such as whole foods, vegetables, and fruits. Follow the Five-A-Day Diet (see page 21). Eating kelp is especially suggested, as this vegetable is highly nutritious. Consuming sweets, and overeating in general, should be avoided. In addition, the nutrients listed in the following table should be part of your daily nutrition plan.

Natural Remedy	Dosage	Comments
Echinacea	*Dried extract:* 300 mg, 3 times daily for 14 days; *Fluid extract:* 1/2 tsp, 3 times daily for 14 days	Appears to lose its immune-boosting properties after a couple of weeks. Therefore, it is best to use this herb for limited periods of treatment.
Multivitamin/ mineral*	See pages 14 to 20.	See pages 14 to 20.
Vitamin A*	25,000 IU daily, for 14 days only	Take with a meal. Can be toxic when taken in large amounts for a long period of time. Be sure to restrict regimen to 14 days, unless a physician directs you otherwise.

Vitamin C*	1,000 mg, 3 times daily	Safe for long-term maintenance.
Vitamin E*	400 IU, daily	Take with a meal. Mixed tocopherols supplying 400 IU of d-alpha tocopherol are preferred. Can be used for long-term maintenance.

* It is important that the discussed nutrients be part of a basic vitamin/mineral regimen so that the total daily amount of each nutrient obtained from both a multivitamin/mineral and other supplements is approximately the dosage indicated above.

Bronchitis

This condition is characterized by an inflammation of the *bronchi*—the breathing tubes that lead to the lungs. It is usually self-limited, with eventual and complete healing and restoration of normal breathing function. Although bronchitis is most often mild, it can be more serious in individuals who have certain illnesses, such as chronic heart or lung diseases. Pneumonia is a critical complication that may follow bronchitis.

Acute bronchitis is most prevalent in winter and may develop after a common cold, flu, or other viral infection. Air pollutants, chilling, fatigue, and malnutrition are factors that play a role in the onset of bronchitis. Symptoms include: persistent coughing; excess accumulation of mucus; chest and back pain; fever; sore throat; and breathing difficulties. Chronic bronchitis differs from the acute form in that it is not an infection. Rather, it is caused by regular irritation of the lungs. Allergies and cigarette smoking are often involved in chronic bronchitis. In the presence of chronic bronchitis, demands on the heart are greater, possibly leading to heart disease.

Do not self-diagnose this condition. Have a doctor confirm that bronchitis is present. Cough suppressants should not be used to regularly treat this condition. However, some OTCs can provide symptomatic relief.

OTC REMEDIES

The products listed in the following chart will help to relieve the symptoms of bronchitis. With the exception of *Benylin Expectorant*, the remedies are analgesics—substances that reduce or relieve pain—and also work to reduce fever. If you have experienced side effects from any nonprescription pain relievers, do not take any analgesic without consulting your doctor. Always read the label before using a product.

OTC Remedy	Dosage	Comments
Acetaminophen *Excedrin Aspirin-Free; Panadol; Tylenol*	325 mg regular strength; generally, 500 mg extra strength	Do not drink alcohol and use products containing acetaminophen. The combination can cause liver damage. Do not take with other analgesics. Some of these products, such as *Tylenol*, are available in regular, junior, and extra strength.

Aspirin (acetylsalicylic acid) *Ascriptin; Bayer; Bufferin; Ecotrin; Empirin; Excedrin Extra Strength*	325 mg regular strength; generally, 500 mg extra strength	If pregnant, consult your doctor before taking products containing aspirin. Do not take products containing aspirin during the last three months of pregnancy. Children and teens should not use products containing aspirin for colds, flus, or chickenpox. Do not take products containing aspirin if you have asthma, stomach problems; gastric ulcers, bleeding problems, or if you are allergic to aspirin.
Benylin Expectorant	Follow product dosage recommendations, which vary with age.	Encourages the loosening and coughing up of respiratory mucus. It is wise to consult with your doctor for proper usage of this medication when it comes to your particular condition.
Ibuprofen *Advil; Arthritis Foundation Ibuprofen; Motrin IB; Nuprin*	200 mg	If pregnant, consult your doctor before taking this remedy. Do not take products containing this ingredient during the last three months of pregnancy. Do not take this ingredient if you are allergic to aspirin. Do not take this ingredient with any other analgesics. Consult your doctor before taking this remedy with prescription drugs.
Ketoprofen *Orudis KT*	12.5 mg	Same comments as Ibuprofen.
Naproxen sodium *Aleve*	220 mg	If pregnant, consult your doctor before taking this remedy. Do not take products containing this ingredient during the last three months of pregnancy.

> Do not take this ingredient
> with any other analgesics.
> Consult your doctor before
> taking this remedy with
> prescription drugs.

When used responsibly, acetaminophen, aspirin, ibuprofen, ketoprofen, and naproxen sodium are safe and effective. Look for single-ingredient products. If you have questions or concerns regarding the safety and effectiveness of any product, consult your doctor or pharmacist.

NATURAL REMEDIES

To relieve the symptoms of bronchitis naturally, drink plenty of liquids, such as water and herbal tea. In addition, echinacea may be of help in restoring health to your respiratory system. Use 300 milligrams of the dried extract, or $1/2$ teaspoon of the fluid extract, three times daily for fourteen days. Echinacea appears to lose its immune-boosting properties after a couple of weeks of use. Therefore, it is best to supplement with this herb only for short periods of treatment.

Bruises

A bruise is an injury of the tissues beneath the skin, while the skin itself is not cut or broken. Common symptoms of bruising include: black and blue marks (caused by blood collecting under the skin); swelling; and pain. Bruising is most often caused by banging into a hard object or from injury during sports activities.

There are also instances when bruising is an indication of an underlying condition. For example, people with *hemophilia*—a disease in which the blood does not clot and the individual can bleed profusely from a tiny injury—bruise easily. Overuse of anticlotting drugs can contribute to bruising, as can deficiencies in vitamin C, vitamin K, the bioflavonoids, and rutin (an enzyme). In addition, anemia, malnutrition, and excess weight may play a role in a person's tendency to bruise. People who bruise easily and consistently should consult a physician.

OTC REMEDIES

The products listed in the first section of the following chart are analgesics—substances that reduce or relieve pain. If you have experienced side effects from any nonprescription pain relievers, do not take any of these remedies without consulting your doctor. The products suggested in the second part are topical remedies, to be applied to the area of the bruise. Always read the label before using any product.

OTC Remedy	Application/Dosage	Comments
Oral Pain-Relieving Medications		
Acetaminophen *Excedrin Aspirin-Free; Panadol; Tylenol*	325 mg regular strength; generally, 500 mg extra strength	Do not drink alcohol and use products containing acetaminophen. The combination can cause liver damage. Do not take with other analgesics. Some of these products, such as *Tylenol,* are available in regular, junior, and extra strength.

Aspirin (acetylsalicylic acid) *Ascriptin; Bayer; Bufferin; Ecotrin; Empirin; Excedrin Extra Strength*	325 mg regular strength; generally, 500 mg extra strength	If pregnant, consult your doctor before taking products containing aspirin. Do not take products containing aspirin during the last three months of pregnancy. Children and teens should not use products containing aspirin for colds, flus, or chickenpox. Do not take products containing aspirin if you have asthma, stomach problems, gastric ulcers, bleeding problems, or if you are allergic to aspirin.
Ibuprofen *Advil; Arthritis Foundation Ibuprofen; Motrin IB; Nuprin*	200 mg	If pregnant, consult your doctor before taking this remedy. Do not take products containing this ingredient during the last three months of pregnancy. Do not take this ingredient if you are allergic to aspirin. Do not take this ingredient with any other analgesics. Consult your doctor before taking this remedy with prescription drugs.
Ketoprofen *Orudis KT*	12.5 mg	Same comments as Ibuprofen.
Naproxen sodium *Aleve*	220 mg	If pregnant, consult your doctor before taking this remedy. Do not take products containing this ingredient during the last three months of pregnancy. Do not take this ingredient with any other analgesics. Consult your doctor before taking this remedy with prescription drugs.

Topical Products		
Bengay Pain-Relieving Ointment/Cream	As directed on label.	Available in original ointment and a greaseless cream. Do not apply to broken or irritated skin.
Capsaicin Capzasin-P Topical Analgesic Creme	As directed on label.	Do not apply to broken or irritated skin.

When used responsibly, acetaminophen, aspirin, ibuprofen, ketoprofen, and naproxen sodium are safe and effective. However, people who bruise easily may want to avoid aspirin or aspirin-containing drugs, as these medications act as blood thinners and make bleeding upon injury more profuse. Look for single-ingredient products. If you have questions or concerns regarding the safety and effectiveness of any product, consult your doctor or pharmacist.

NATURAL REMEDIES

In general, the application of ice to the bruised area for no more than thirty minutes at a time is sufficient to treat this condition. To reduce bruising due to lack of proper nutrition, consume a diet high in vitamin C and the bioflavonoids. Such a diet would include, for example, dark green leafy vegetables, buckwheat, and fresh fruit. The dark green leafy vegetables—such as kale, chard, collards, beets, spinach, watercress, mustard greens, and turnips—also add significant vitamin K to the diet. If preferred, the vegetables can be made into juice. For supplementation, follow the guidelines provided in the chart below.

Natural Remedy	Dosage	Comments
Bioflavonoids	1,000 mg, 3 times daily	Help to strengthen the capillaries to prevent them from breaking easily.
Horse chestnut extract *Venostat*	35 to 70 mg, daily	Rich in specific bioflavonoids and has been shown to strengthen capillaries. It may also increase the tone of veins, which prevents them from expanding to form hemorrhoids. Select an extract standardized to aescin content. Aescin is the active ingredient.
Vitamin C*	1,000 mg, 3 times daily	Safe for long-term maintenance.

* It is important that the discussed nutrients be part of a basic vitamin/mineral regimen so that the total daily amount of each nutrient obtained from both a multivitamin/mineral and other supplements is approximately the dosage indicated above.

Bruxism

This condition, which involves the clenching and grinding of the teeth, is the most common motor abnormality of the oral area. Over time, bruxism erodes and diminishes the teeth. Also, teeth may loosen. An individual with bruxism may not even be aware of the condition. However, friends and family members usually notice it.

A conscious effort must be made to overcome this habitual condition. A physician may prescribe helpful sedatives or minor tranquilizers. Furthermore, a dentist can provide a splint to be worn over the teeth, to prevent grinding. Keep in mind that the use of alcohol frequently worsens bruxism.

OTC REMEDIES

The products listed in the following chart are analgesics—substances that relieve or reduce pain. If you have experienced side effects from any nonprescription pain relievers, do not take any of these remedies without consulting your doctor. Always read the label before using a product.

OTC Remedy	Dosage	Comments
Acetaminophen *Excedrin Aspirin-Free; Panadol; Tylenol*	325 mg regular strength; generally, 500 mg extra strength	Do not drink alcohol and use products containing acetaminophen. The combination can cause liver damage. Do not take with other analgesics. Some of these products, such as *Tylenol,* are available in regular, junior, and extra strength.
Aspirin (acetylsalicylic acid) *Ascriptin; Bayer; Bufferin; Ecotrin; Empirin; Excedrin Extra Strength*	325 mg regular strength; generally, 500 mg extra strength	If pregnant, consult your doctor before taking products containing aspirin. Do not take products containing aspirin during the last three months of pregnancy. Children and teens should not use products containing aspirin for colds, flus, or chickenpox. Do not take products containing aspirin if you have asthma, stomach problems, gastric ulcers, bleeding problems, or if you are allergic to aspirin.

Ibuprofen *Advil;* *Arthritis* *Foundation* *Ibuprofen;* *Motrin IB;* *Nuprin*	200 mg	If pregnant, consult your doctor before taking this remedy. Do not take products containing this ingredient during the last three months of pregnancy. Do not take this ingredient if you are allergic to aspirin. Do not take this ingredient with any other analgesics. Consult your doctor before taking this remedy with prescription drugs.
Ketoprofen *Orudis KT*	12.5 mg	Same comments as Ibuprofen.
Naproxen sodium *Aleve*	220 mg	If pregnant, consult your doctor before taking this remedy. Do not take products containing this ingredient during the last three months of pregnancy. Do not take this ingredient with any other analgesics. Consult your doctor before taking this remedy with prescription drugs.

When used responsibly, acetaminophen, aspirin, ibuprofen, ketoprofen, and naproxen sodium are safe and effective. Look for single-ingredient products. If you have questions or concerns regarding the safety and effectiveness of any product, consult your doctor or pharmacist.

NATURAL REMEDIES

Stress management and relaxation techniques can be helpful and can reduce the need for medication.

Biofeedback is another alternative approach that may be very effective. Also, avoid eating sugar six hours before bed, and limit intake of colas and processed foods. Finally, the recommendations in the chart below may be of help.

Natural Remedy	Dosage	Comments
Calcium tablet	1 chewable tablet at bedtime	May help to reduce contractions of jaw muscles. Be sure to attain up to 1,200 mg of total calcium intake daily, including that received from food sources.
Multivitamin/mineral	See pages 14 to 20.	See pages 14 to 20. A good multivitamin/mineral will help maintain muscle and bone health.

Burns

Tissue injury by burning can be caused by thermal, chemical, or electrical contact. Minor burns can usually be self-treated. Some first- and second-degree burns require outpatient treatment by a health-care professional. All third-degree burns require the immediate attention of a physician.

The severity of the burn is determined by: the quantity of tissue involved; the amount of body surface burned; and the depth of the burn. First-degree burns are characterized by redness and sensitivity to touch and moistness; second-degree burns by redness and, sometimes, blisters; and third-degree burns by destruction of the entire thickness of the skin, as well as of the underlying muscle. Third-degree burns are usually not sensitive to touch, as the nerves have been severely damaged.

OTC REMEDIES

The products listed in the first section of the following table are analgesics—substances that relieve or reduce pain. If you have experienced side effects from any nonprescription pain relievers, do not take any of these remedies without consulting your doctor. The second section of the table lists topical products that should be applied directly to the burned area. Always read the label before using a product.

OTC Remedy	Dosage	Comments
Oral Pain-Relieving Medications		
Acetaminophen *Excedrin Aspirin-Free; Panadol; Tylenol*	325 mg regular strength; generally, 500 mg extra strength	Do not drink alcohol and use products containing acetaminophen. The combination can cause liver damage. Do not take with other analgesics. Some of these products, such as *Tylenol,* are available in regular, junior, and extra strength.
Aspirin (acetylsalicylic acid) *Ascriptin; Bayer; Bufferin; Ecotrin; Empirin; Excedrin Extra Strength*	325 mg regular strength; generally, 500 mg extra strength	If pregnant, consult your doctor before taking products containing aspirin. Do not take products containing aspirin during the last three months of pregnancy. Children and teens should not use products containing aspirin for colds, flus, or chickenpox. Do not take products containing aspirin if you have asthma, stomach problems, gastric ulcers, bleeding problems, or if you are allergic to aspirin.

Ibuprofen *Advil;* *Arthritis* *Foundation* *Ibuprofen;* *Motrin IB; Nuprin*	200 mg	If pregnant, consult your doctor before taking this remedy. Do not take products containing this ingredient during the last three months of pregnancy. Do not take this ingredient if you are allergic to aspirin. Do not take this ingredient with any other analgesics. Consult your doctor before taking this remedy with prescription drugs.
Ketoprofen *Orudis KT*	12.5 mg	Same comments as Ibuprofen.
Naproxen sodium *Aleve*	220 mg	If pregnant, consult your doctor before taking this remedy. Do not take products containing this ingredient during the last three months of pregnancy. Do not take this ingredient with any other analgesics. Consult your doctor before taking this remedy with prescription drugs.

Topical Products

A & D Ointment	As directed on label.	Skin astringent, protectant, and antiseptic (kills microorganisms).
Americaine Topical Anesthetic Spray and First Aid Ointment	As directed on label.	Temporarily blocks the pain messages sent from the skin to the brain. No common side effects. Further skin irritation (possibly including hives) is unusual.
Bactine Antiseptic Anesthetic First Aid Liquid	As directed on label.	Reduces inflammation, kills bacteria, and temporarily blocks pain messages sent from the skin to the brain. No common side effects.

		Further skin irritation is unusual. Do not use if you are allergic to cortisone products.
Bactine First Aid Antibiotic Plus Anesthetic Ointment	As directed on label.	Same comments as *Bactine Antiseptic Anesthetic First Aid Liquid.*
BiCozene Creme	As directed on label.	Topical anti-infective. No common side effects. Further skin irritation is unusual.
Mycitracin Maximum Strength Triple Antibiotic First Aid Ointment	As directed on label.	Kills bacteria. No common side effects. Further skin irritation is unusual. Do not use if you are allergic to any of the following antibiotics or related substances: chloramphenicol; gentamicin; mupirocin; neomycin; polymyxins.
Mycitracin Plus Pain Reliever	As directed on label.	Same comments as *Mycitracin Maximum Strength Triple Antibiotic First Aid Ointment.* Also temporarily relieves pain by blocking pain messages sent from the skin to the brain.
Neosporin Ointment	As directed on label.	Also available in *Plus Maximum Strength.* Same comments as *Mycitracin Maximum Strength Triple Antibiotic First Aid Ointment.*

When used responsibly, acetaminophen, aspirin, ibuprofen, ketoprofen, and naproxen sodium are safe and effective. Look for single-ingredient products. If you have questions or concerns regarding the safety and effectiveness of any product, consult your doctor or pharmacist.

NATURAL REMEDIES

If you get a minor burn, before using ointments or salves, apply cold to reduce pain and swelling. Ice water or a cold compress is the best remedy to use immediately after the burn occurs. Then, for local treatment of first- and second-degree burns, apply aloe vera gel directly to the affected area. Placing cool applications of calendula or chamomile tea on the burn can also be soothing. In addition to local treatment, the following vitamin and mineral supplements may assist in the healing of first- and second-degree burns that cover more than a small area of the body.

Natural Remedy	Dosage	Comments
Vitamin A*	*During first week:* 50,000 IU, daily; *Thereafter:* 25,000 IU, daily	Take with a meal. Can be toxic when taken in large amounts for a long period of time. Be sure to restrict regimen to the dosage recommended, unless a physician directs you otherwise.
Vitamin C*	5,000 to 10,000 mg, daily	Safe for long-term maintenance.
Vitamin E*	400 to 800 IU, daily	Take with a meal. Mixed tocopherols supplying 400 IU of d-alpha tocopherol are preferred. Can be used for long-term maintenance.

| Zinc* | 30 mg, daily | Take with a meal. Doses in excess of 100 mg can depress immune function. |

* It is important that the discussed nutrients be part of a basic vitamin/mineral regimen so that the total daily amount of each nutrient obtained from both a multivitamin/mineral and other supplements is approximately the dosage indicated above.

Bursitis

This condition is characterized by an acute or chronic inflammation of a *bursa*—a sac-like cavity filled with fluid and located at tissue sites in the body where friction occurs, such as at joints, tendons, muscles, and bones. Bursae facilitate normal body movements and minimize friction between moving body parts. Bursitis can result from trauma, chronic overuse, arthritis, calcium deposits, certain foods, airborne allergies, and infection. This condition most frequently affects the shoulders, hips, and elbows. In fact, when individuals suffer from a "frozen shoulder" or "tennis elbow," they have bursitis.

Common symptoms of bursitis are tenderness and acute pain in the affected area. Successful treatment involves elimination of the cause of the injury. Sometimes an underlying infection must be cleared up. On occasion, calcium deposits will require removal by surgery.

OTC REMEDIES

The products listed in the following chart are analgesics—substances that reduce or relieve pain. If you have experienced side effects from any nonprescription pain relievers, do not take any of these remedies without consulting your doctor. Always read the label before using a product.

OTC Remedy	Dosage	Comments
Acetaminophen *Excedrin Aspirin-Free; Panadol; Tylenol*	325 mg regular strength; generally, 500 mg extra strength	Do not drink alcohol and use products containing acetaminophen. The combination can cause liver damage. Do not take with other analgesics. Some of these products, such as *Tylenol,* are available in regular, junior, and extra strength.
Aspirin (acetylsalicylic acid) *Ascriptin; Bayer; Bufferin; Ecotrin; Empirin; Excedrin Extra Strength*	325 mg regular strength; generally, 500 mg extra strength	If pregnant, consult your doctor before taking products containing aspirin. Do not take products containing aspirin during the last three months of pregnancy. Children and teens should not use products containing aspirin for colds, flus, or chickenpox. Do not take products containing aspirin if you have asthma, stomach problems, gastric ulcers, bleeding problems, or if you are allergic to aspirin.
Ibuprofen *Advil; Arthritis Foundation Ibuprofen; Motrin IB; Nuprin*	200 mg	If pregnant, consult your doctor before taking this remedy. Do not take products containing this ingredient during the last three months of pregnancy. Do not take this ingredient if you are allergic to aspirin. Do not take this ingredient with any other analgesics. Consult your doctor before

		taking this remedy with prescription drugs.
Ketoprofen *Orudis KT*	12.5 mg	Same comments as Ibuprofen.
Naproxen sodium *Aleve*	220 mg	If pregnant, consult your doctor before taking this remedy. Do not take products containing this ingredient during the last three months of pregnancy. Do not take this ingredient with any other analgesics. Consult your doctor before taking this remedy with prescription drugs.

When used responsibly, acetaminophen, aspirin, ibuprofen, ketoprofen, and naproxen sodium are safe and effective. Look for single-ingredient products. If you have questions or concerns regarding the safety and effectiveness of any product, consult your doctor or pharmacist.

NATURAL REMEDIES

The table below offers supplementation recommendations that should help to relieve the discomforts of bursitis. Keep in mind that no matter what remedy you use, treatment of bursitis should be monitored by a physician so that the condition does not become chronic. Some individuals find injections of vitamins B_3 and B_{12} effective. Consult a nutritionally-oriented physician for more information.

Natural Remedy	Dosage	Comments
Boswellia	400 mg	Look for a standardized extract. A resin extracted from a tree in India. It has been shown to reduce inflammation without the side effects common to OTC anti-inflammatories. Usage of boswellia should be monitored by a physician.
Multivitamin/ mineral with antioxidants	See pages 14 to 20.	See pages 14 to 20. Be sure that your regimen provides 1,200 mg of calcium and 400 to 600 mg of magnesium daily.

Candidiasis

See also Vaginitis; Yeast Infections.

Candidiasis is a yeast-like infection caused by a fungus called *Candida albicans*. It can infect the genital tract, mouth, throat, and intestine. When the infection occurs in the mouth or throat, it is called *thrush*. Candidiasis is increasing in frequency among women. It is not commonly sexually transmitted.

Candida albicans usually spreads from the patient's skin or intestinal flora. The widespread use of broadspectrum antibiotics and oral contraceptives is involved in the increased prevalence of candidiasis. Infected men are generally symptomless. Women develop obvious symptoms—vaginitis, with a copious amount of white, cheesy discharge and severe itching. Other symptoms include constipation; diarrhea; abdominal pain; colitis; sore throat; canker sores; and kidney and bladder pain. An infected mother may pass the infection to her newborn child.

There is no easy way to detect this condition. Women who have infants and who care for infants should keep in mind how easy it is to transmit this fungus to babies. Also, diabetics are at greater risk for this condition than the general population.

OTC REMEDIES

The products listed in the following table can provide symptomatic relief from candidiasis. Always read the label before using a product.

OTC Remedy	Application	Comments
Gyne-Lotrimin Vaginal Cream/ Inserts/ Combination Pack	As directed on label.	Kills fungus cells. No common side effects. Irritation, burning, itching, and increased discharge in the vaginal area due to use of these products are uncommon. Do not use if you have a liver disorder.
Mycelex-7 Vaginal Cream/ Inserts/ Combination Pack	As directed on label.	Same comments as *Gyne-Lotrimin* products.
Miconazole nitrate *Monistat 7 Vaginal Cream/Inserts*	As directed on label.	Same comments as *Gyne-Lotrimin* products.

Long-term or recurring problems with candidiasis require a conventional or naturopathic physician's help in diagnosing the underlying causes and in organizing a helpful dietary plan. But for occasional outbreaks, OTCs work well.

NATURAL REMEDIES

There are several natural approaches that help to relieve the symptoms of candidiasis. Consume a diet low in fat, sugar, refined carbohydrates, and alcohol. A high-sugar diet encourages the overgrowth of the candida organisms. Eat yogurt or take acidophilus capsules, as instructed in the following table.

In truth, for infrequent infections, OTC drugs are the best choice. But if your problem is recurrent, herbs taken for immune maintenance may be helpful. The following table offers a possible program. However, it is important to consult your health-care professional concerning a regimen that is most effective for your individual situation. *It is important to note that while certain herbal regimens help maintain a healthy immune system, people with autoimmune illnesses, such as lupus, and those with progressive diseases, such as tuberculosis and multiple sclerosis, should not use herbs for the immune system without consulting their physicians.*

Natural Remedy	Dosage	Comments
Acidophilus *(Lactobacillus acidophilus)*	3 capsules or $\frac{1}{4}$ tsp powder, 1 to 3 times daily	Friendly bacteria that help maintain bacterial balance. Purchase products that have been refrigerated, to ensure potency.
Astragalus	*During infection:* (3) 500-mg capsules/tablets, 3 times daily;	A Chinese remedy used for thousands of years; a proven immune stimulant.

	For maintenance: (3) 500-mg capsules/tablets daily	
Cat's claw	20 to 60 mg, daily	Use standardized extract. Among other functions, it increases white blood cell activity and helps to clean the intestinal tract. Pregnant and lactating women should not use this herb.
Siberian ginseng *(Eleutherococcus senticosus)*	300 to 400 mg, daily	Use standardized extract to help balance body systems.
Garlic	1 clove daily, or equivalent dosage in capsules/tablets	Enteric coated tablets standardized to allicin potential are preferred.
Green tea	3 to 4 cups (decaffeinated) tea daily, or the equivalent in capsules/tablets that provide over 70-percent polyphenols	One of the best immune boosters and antiaging foods; has been found to reduce the risk of certain types of cancer.
Shiitake	1,000 mg LEM, daily	LEM (lentinan edodes mycelium) is the most potent extract of the shiitake mushroom.

Canker Sores

Canker sores are acute, painful ulcers—*apthous ulcers*—found on the mouth, either singly or in groups. They may appear on the lips, tongue, gums, or inside cheeks. The size of the sores varies greatly, from barely noticeable to quite large. Canker sores usually appear suddenly and are gone within four to twenty days.

The cause of canker sores is not definitively known, but a localized immune reaction is suspected. Deficiencies of iron, vitamin B_{12}, and folic acid may also be involved. In addition, stress, allergies, poor dental hygiene, and fatigue may all play a role in the development of canker sores. They are contagious, and women experience this condition more frequently than men.

OTC REMEDIES

The products listed in the following table provide symptomatic relief from canker sores. Always read the label before using a product.

OTC Remedy	Application	Comments
Herpicin-L Cold Sore Lip Balm with SPF 15 Sunscreen	Apply to lips, as directed on label.	Provides a protective coating for the lips.
Orajel Mouth-Aid Cold/Canker Sore Medicine	Apply to sore, as directed on label.	Temporarily blocks pain messages sent from affected area to the brain. No common side effects. Increased irritation from use of this product is unusual.
Orajel Perioseptic	Apply to sore, as directed on label.	Topical antiseptic (kills microorganisms).

NATURAL REMEDIES

Discontinue activities that can spread canker sores until the condition is clearly resolved. In addition, avoid all of the following: chewing gums; lozenges;

mouthwashes; smoking; coffee; citrus fruits; processed and sugary foods and sweets. Making a few changes to your diet can balance the alkalinity and acidity levels in your body and, therefore, help you to avoid this condition. Add cottage cheese, yogurt, and buttermilk to your diet; include onions in your salads. For two weeks after an outbreak, avoid alcohol and decrease your intake of meat and fish.

Some individuals find that iron supplemenation is helpful, as iron deficiency has been identified with recurrent mouth ulcers. However, this treatment requires a doctor's guidance. Similarly, large doses (300+ milligrams) of vitamin B_1 may be helpful, but must be managed under a doctor's supervision. The following table suggests several supplementation options that do not need to be monitored by a physician.

Natural Remedy	Dosage/Application	Comments
Acidophilus (Lactobacillus acidophilus)	4 capsules/tablets, 3 times daily	Purchase products that have been refrigerated, to ensure potency.
Chamomile tea	As often as needed.	May provide a soothing effect.
Myrrh tincture	Topical application, 2 to 3 times daily	Antiseptic (kills microorganisms) and disinfectant.
Vitamin-B complex*	50 mg of all B-vitamins, daily	A high incidence of vitamin-B deficiency has been identified in people with recurrent mouth ulcers.

* It is important that the discussed nutrients be part of a basic vitamin/mineral regimen so that the total daily amount of each nutrient obtained from both a multivitamin/mineral and other supplements is approximately the dosage indicated above.

Cholesterol

See High Cholesterol.

Chronic Fatigue Syndrome (CFS)

Chronic fatigue syndrome occurs mainly among adults between the ages of twenty and forty. Twice as many women suffer from CFS as men. Some of the symptoms include: extreme fatigue; loss of appetite; sore throat; fever; swollen lymph glands; mood swings; anxiety; depression; irritability; sleep disturbances; difficulty concentrating; muscular and joint aches; and headaches. CFS often resembles the flu or other viral infections. It is sometimes misdiagnosed as as a psychosomatic or hypochondriacal complaint.

CFS is not life-threatening, but it is debilitating and interferes with a person's ability to live a happy, productive life. Although some people within the medical field firmly believe that CFS is caused by the *Epstein-Barr virus* (EBV), the medical jury is not in yet. Epstein-Barr virus is also linked to mononucleosis. The Centers for Disease Control estimate that tens of thousands of Americans are infected with EBV. The virus is contagious and can be transmitted through kissing, coughing, sexual contact, and sharing food.

OTC REMEDIES

The products listed in the following chart are analgesics—substances that relieve or reduce pain. These products also combat fever. If you have experienced side effects from any nonprescription pain relievers, do not take any of these remedies without consulting your doctor. Always read the label before using a product.

OTC Remedy	Dosage	Comments
Acetaminophen *Excedrin Aspirin-Free; Panadol; Tylenol*	325 mg regular strength; generally, 500 mg extra strength	Do not drink alcohol and use products containing acetaminophen. The combination can cause liver damage. Do not take with other analgesics. Some of these products, such as *Tylenol,* are available in regular, junior, and extra strength.
Aspirin (acetylsalicylic acid) *Ascriptin; Bayer; Bufferin; Ecotrin; Empirin; Excedrin Extra Strength*	325 mg regular strength; generally, 500 mg extra strength	If pregnant, consult your doctor before taking products containing aspirin. Do not take products containing aspirin during the last three months of pregnancy. Children and teens should not use products containing aspirin for colds, flus, or chickenpox. Do not take products containing aspirin if you have asthma, stomach problems, gastric ulcers, bleeding problems, or if you are allergic to aspirin.
Ibuprofen *Advil; Arthritis Foundation Ibuprofen; Motrin IB; Nuprin*	200 mg	If pregnant, consult your doctor before taking this remedy. Do not take products containing this ingredient during the last three months of pregnancy. Do not take this ingredient if

		you are allergic to aspirin. Do not take this ingredient with any other analgesics. Consult your doctor before taking this remedy with prescription drugs.
Ketoprofen *Orudis KT*	12.5 mg	Same comments as Ibuprofen.
Naproxen sodium *Aleve*	220 mg	If pregnant, consult your doctor before taking this remedy. Do not take products containing this ingredient during the last three months of pregnancy. Do not take this ingredient with any other analgesics. Consult your doctor before taking this remedy with prescription drugs.

When used responsibly, acetaminophen, aspirin, ibuprofen, ketoprofen, and naproxen sodium are safe and effective. Look for single-ingredient products. If you have questions or concerns regarding the safety and effectiveness of any product, consult your doctor or pharmacist.

NATURAL REMEDIES

As with many conditions, diet can play a role in alleviating the symptoms of chronic fatigue syndrome. Eating lots of whole, pure foods, including raw vegetables and fresh juices, is very important. Eliminating sugar, alcohol, caffeine (coffee, tea, soft drinks), white flour products, and processed, fried, and junk foods can be very effective. In addition, food allergies can sometimes trigger symptoms identical to those of CFS. Try the "elimination/rotation/add-back diet" outlined in the entry on food allergy (page 188) to determine if you may be suffering from an allergic reaction to certain foods. Finally, the following chart lists several natural substances that are helpful in combatting the effects of CFS.

Natural Remedy	Dosage	Comments
CoQ$_{10}$ (coenzyme Q$_{10}$, also called ubiquinone)	75 mg, daily	Some people respond rapidly to this nutrient's ability to increase energy output. It is most known for its cardiovascular benefits.
Multivitamin/ mineral*	See pages 14 to 20.	See pages 14 to 20.
NADH *ENADA*	10 mg, daily	A stable form of the nutrient NADH that has been shown to alleviate some symptoms associated with CFS.
Siberian ginseng (*Eleutherococcus senticosus*)	200 mg, daily	Try a standardized extract containing more than 1-percent eleutheroside E.
Vitamin C*	1,000 mg, 3 times daily	Safe for long-term maintenance.
Vitamin E*	400 IU, daily	Take after a meal. Mixed tocopherols supplying 400 IU of d-alpha tocopherol are preferred. Can be used for long-term maintenance.

* It is important that the discussed nutrients be part of a basic vitamin/mineral regimen so that the total daily amount of each nutrient obtained from both a multivitamin/mineral and other supplements is approximately the dosage indicated above.

Cold Sores

This condition, also called "fever blisters," is caused by the herpes simplex virus I. Cold sores usually occur around the mouth, although they can also form in the area of other mucous membranes. Generally, tenderness around a small bump is the first sign of an emerging cold sore. Eventually, a blister forms and there may be tenderness in a wider area. In addition, some cold sores ooze pus. They can last anywhere from a few days to three weeks.

Cold sores are extremely contagious. They often accompany fevers, infections, and colds. Stress, overexposure to sun and wind, menstruation, and lowered immune-system functioning also play roles in the appearance of cold sores, which develop three to ten days after exposure to the causative factor. People with allergies may experience episodes of cold sores more frequently. Avoid activities that can spread these sores until the condition is clearly resolved.

OTC REMEDIES

The chart below lists several products that offer symptomatic relief from cold sores. Always read the label before using a product.

OTC Remedy	Dosage	Comments
Herpecin-L Cold Sore Lip Balm with SPF 15 Sunscreen	Apply to lips, as directed on label.	Provides a protective coating.

| *Orajel Mouth-Aid Cold/Canker Sore Medicine* | Apply to sore, as directed on the label. | Temporarily blocks pain messages sent from affected area to the brain. No common side effects. Increased irritation from use of this product is unusual. |

NATURAL REMEDIES

Lysine and arginine are naturally occurring amino acids. They sometimes "compete" with each other. For example, the herpes virus is nurtured by arginine, but lysine can block the availability of arginine and thereby prevent the virus from becoming active. So, to help prevent cold sores, refrain from eating foods that are high in arginine and/or low in lysine, such as: chocolate, almonds, peanuts, cashews, cottonseed oil, corn, wheat, oats, grains, and gelatin. Also, keep in mind that sun exposure can trigger an outbreak of cold sores in some individuals.

The best strategy is to strengthen the immune system so that the body can resist the virus that causes the outbreak. To boost your immune system, consume raw vegetables, yogurt, and soured products. Get plenty of rest and regular exercise. The following chart contains further instruction. Consult a nutritionist for advice on your individual situation. *It is important to note that while certain herbal regimens help maintain a healthy immune system, people with autoimmune illnesses, such as lupus, and those with progressive diseases, such as tuberculosis and multiple sclerosis, should not use herbs for the immune system without consulting their physicians.*

Natural Remedy	Dosage	Comments
Astragalus	*During infection:* (3) 500-mg capsules/tablets, 3 times daily; *For maintenance:* (3) 500-mg capsules/tablets, daily	A Chinese remedy used for thousands of years; a proven immune stimulant.
Cat's claw	20 to 60 mg, daily	Use standardized extract. Pregnant and lactating women should not use this herb.
Garlic	1 clove daily, or equivalent dosage in capsules/tablets	Enteric coated tablets standardized to allicin potential are preferred.
Green tea	3 to 4 cups (decaffeinated) tea daily, or equivalent in capsules/tablets that provide over 70-percent polyphenols	One of the best immune boosters and antiaging foods. Green tea has been found to reduce the risk of certain types of cancer.
Multivitamin/ mineral*	See pages 14 to 20.	See pages 14 to 20.
Lysine	*At first sign of outbreak:* 1,000 mg, 3 times daily; *For maintenance:* 500 mg, 2 times daily	A natural amino acid that competes with the arginine and helps to deny it access to the virus.
Shiitake	1,000 mg LEM, daily, for maintenance	LEM (lentinan edodes mycelium) is an extract of the shiitake mushroom that is most potent.
Siberian ginseng (*Eleutherococcus senticosus*)	300 to 400 mg, daily, for maintenance	Use standardized extract containing more than 1-percent eleutheroside E.

| Zinc* | *For first two days of infection:* 15 mg, 4 times daily; *For maintenance:* 15 mg, 2 times daily | Take with a meal. Doses in excess of 100 mg can depress immune function and cause an imbalance in levels of other minerals. Check the amount of zinc in your multivitamin/mineral before supplementing with additional zinc. |

* It is important that the discussed nutrients be part of a basic vitamin/mineral regimen so that the total daily amount of each nutrient obtained from both a multivitamin/mineral and other supplements is approximately the dosage indicated above.

Colds and Coughs

The common cold is an acute viral infection of the respiratory tract that usually does not involve a fever. There is generally inflammation of all airways—nose, sinuses, throat, larynx, trachea, and bronchi of the lungs. Symptoms of a cold appear within one to three days of exposure to the virus. Included among these symptoms are: headache; sneezing; watery eyes; running nose; congestion; coughing; difficulty breathing; and aches and pains.

About 30 to 50 percent of all colds are caused by one of the more than a hundred kinds of rhinoviruses known to medicine. Spring, summer, and autumn colds are almost always due to the picornavirus; late autumn and winter colds are associated with the myxovirus, paramyxovirus, and pneumovirus. There is no cure for the common cold, but there are both prevention and treatment measures that you can take. If there is congestion in the chest, a fever above 102° F for more than three days, and/or other serious symptoms, see a doctor.

Often, the cough that accompanies a cold is your body's way of ridding itself of pathogens. Therefore, if tolerable, it is good to let your body do what it has to do—don't suppress your cough. However, if you cannot get adequate sleep or if your physician directs you to take a cough medicine to relieve some of your discomfort, there are plenty of products on the market.

In some cases, chest congestion is the problem. Too much mucus has built up and settled in the respiratory system. Expectorants can help to loosen the congestion and allow you to cough some of the mucus out of your lung area.

OTC REMEDIES

In the following table, the products listed under acetaminophen, aspirin, ibuprofen, ketoprofen, and naproxen sodium are analgesics—substances that relieve or reduce pain. These products also combat fever. If you have experienced side effects from any nonprescription pain relievers, do not take any of these remedies without consulting your doctor. The chart is further categorized to recommend products for general cold symptoms (which include congestion, watery eyes, sneezing, etc.); cold and cough symptoms; cough only; and nasal congestion. Always read the label before using a product.

OTC Remedy	Dosage	Comments
Oral Pain-Relieving Medications		
Acetaminophen *Excedrin Aspirin-Free; Panadol; Tylenol*	325 mg regular strength; generally, 500 mg extra strength	Do not drink alcohol and use products containing acetaminophen. The combination can cause liver damage. Do not take with other analgesics. Some of these products, such as *Tylenol,* are available in regular, Junior, and extra strength.
Aspirin (acetylsalicylic acid) *Ascriptin; Bayer; Bufferin; Ecotrin; Empirin; Excedrin Extra Strength*	325 mg regular strength; generally, 500 mg extra strength	If pregnant, consult your doctor before taking products containing aspirin. Do not take products containing aspirin during the last three months of pregnancy. Children and teens should not use products containing aspirin for colds, flus, or chickenpox. Do not take products containing aspirin if you have asthma, stomach problems, gastric ulcers, bleeding problems, or if you are allergic to aspirin.
Ibuprofen *Advil; Arthritis Foundation Ibuprofen; Motrin IB; Nuprin*	200 mg	If pregnant, consult your doctor before taking this remedy. Do not take products containing this ingredient during the last three months of pregnancy. Do not take this ingredient if you are allergic to aspirin. Do not take this ingredient with any other analgesics. Consult your doctor before taking this remedy with prescription drugs.
Ketoprofen *Orudis KT*	12.5 mg	Same comments as Ibuprofen.

| **Naproxen sodium** *Aleve* | 220 mg | • If pregnant, consult your doctor before taking this remedy. Do not take products containing this ingredient during the last three months of pregnancy. Do not take this ingredient with any other analgesics. Consult your doctor before taking this remedy with prescription drugs. |

General Cold Symptom Medications

| **Acetaminophen** *Coricidin "D"; Coricidin Tablets; Drixoral Cold & Flu Extended-Release Tablets; Theraflu Flu & Cold Medicine; Tylenol Severe Allergy Medicine Caplets; Benadryl Allergy Sinus Headache* | 325 mg regular strength; follow manufacturer's dosage instructions for each product. | Do not drink alcohol and use products containing acetaminophen. The combination can cause liver damage. Do not take with other analgesics. |
| **Aspirin** (acetylsalicylic acid) *Alka-Seltzer Plus Cold Medicine* | 325 mg regular strength | If pregnant, consult your doctor before taking products containing aspirin. Do not take products containing aspirin during the last three months of pregnancy. Children and teens should not use products containing aspirin for colds, flus, or chickenpox. Do not take products containing aspirin if you have asthma, stomach problems, gastric ulcers, bleeding problems, or if you are allergic to aspirin. |

!buprofen Advil Cold & Sinus; Motrin IB Cold & Sinus	200 mg	If pregnant, consult your doctor before taking this remedy. Do not take products containing this ingredient during the last three months of pregnancy. Do not take this ingredient if you are allergic to aspirin. Do not take this ingredient with any other analgesics. Consult your doctor before taking this remedy with prescription drugs.
Actifed	As directed on label.	May cause some drowsiness and/or dryness of the mucous membranes. Look for a non-drowsy formula or take necessary precautions. Maintain fluid intake.
Benadryl Allergy Liquid/ Tablets/Kapseals	As directed on label.	Same comments as *Actifed*.
Dimetapp Tablets/ Liqui-gels/Elixir	As directed on label.	May cause some headache, drowsiness, and/or dryness/ stinging of the mucous membranes. Look for a non-drowsy formula or take necessary precautions. Maintain fluid intake.
Drixoral Cold & Allergy Sustained-Action Tablets	As directed on label.	Same comments as *Actifed*.
Efidac 24	As directed on label.	Same comments as *Actifed*.
Neo-Synephrine Nasal Sprays/Drops	As directed on label.	This product is available in various strengths and in pediatric formula. No common side effects. Dryness and irritation of the nasal passages occur only infrequently.

PediaCare Cold-Allergy Chewable Tablets	As directed on label.	Same comments as *Actifed*.
Sudafed Caplets/ Tablets/Liquid	As directed on label.	Available in various strengths and formulas, among which is a children's liquid. See above comments for Acetaminophen, as some formulas contain that ingredient. Same comments as *Actifed*.
Tavist-1 Tablets	As directed on label.	Same comments as *Actifed*.
Tavist-D Tablets	As directed on label.	Same comments as *Actifed*.
Triaminic Syrup/Tablets	As directed on label.	Same comments as *Actifed*.
Triaminic-12 Tablets	As directed on label.	Same comments as *Actifed*.

Cold and Cough Medications

Acetaminophen *Children's Tylenol Cold Multi-Symptom Chewable Tablets/ Liquid; Children's Tylenol Cold Plus Cough Multi-Symptom Chewable Tablets/ Liquid; Comtrex Maximum Strength Multi Symptom Cold Reliever; Contac Severe Cold & Flu Non-Drowsy Caplets; Theraflu Cold & Cough Medicine; Tylenol Cold Medicine Multi Symptom Formula Tablets/Caplets*	325 mg regular strength; follow manufacturer's dosage instructions for each product	Do not drink alcohol and use products containing acetaminophen. The combination can cause liver damage. Do not take with other analgesics. Some of these products are available in several forms. For example, *Theraflu* is available in maximum-strength formula for nighttime use, and in maximum-strength non-drowsy formula.

Aspirin (acetylsalicylic acid) *Alka-Seltzer Plus Cold & Cough Medicine*	325 mg regular strength	If pregnant, consult your doctor before taking products containing aspirin. Do not take products containing aspirin during the last three months of pregnancy. Children and teens should not use products containing aspirin for colds, flus, or chickenpox. Do not take products containing aspirin if you have asthma, stomach problems, gastric ulcers, bleeding problems, or if you are allergic to aspirin.
PediaCare Cough-Cold Liquid/Chewable Tablets	As directed on label.	Also available in *NightRest* liquid formula. Can cause some drowsiness, dizziness, and nasal/oral/throat dryness. Take necessary precautions and maintain fluid intake. More severe adverse reactions are rare.
Robitussin-CF	As directed on label.	No common side effects. Minor stomach and head discomfort, diarrhea, dizziness, sleepiness, nasal/oral dryness, and rashes occur in some individuals, but are unusual. More severe adverse reactions are rare.
Robitussin-DM	As directed on label.	No common side effects. Minor stomach discomfort, diarrhea, dizziness, sleepiness, and rashes occur in some individuals, but are unusual. More severe adverse reactions are rare.
Robitussin Cold and Cough Formulas	As directed on label.	Available in maximum-strength and pediatric formulas. Same comments as *Robitussin-DM*.
Vicks 44d Dry Hacking Cough & Head Congestion	As directed on label.	Available in pediatric formula as well. Same comments as *Robitussin-DM*.

Vicks Children's Nyquil Cold/Cough Relief	As directed on label.	Same comments as *Robitussin-DM*.
Vicks Vaporub/Cream	As directed on label.	Menthol action is cooling and soothing.

Cough Medication

Benylin Cough Suppressant	As directed on label.	Available in different formulas, including adult strength and pediatric. Also available in *NightRest* liquid formula. Can cause some drowsiness, dizziness, and nasal/oral/throat dryness. Take necessary precautions and maintain fluid intake. Do not take for a persistent or chronic cough, or if you have excessive phlegm, unless otherwise directed by a doctor.
Benylin Expectorant	As directed on label.	No common side effects. Minor stomach discomfort, diarrhea, dizziness, sleepiness, and rashes occur in some individuals, but are unusual. Do not take for a persistent or chronic cough, if you have excessive phlegm, or If you have heart disease, high blood pressure, thyroid disease, diabetes, or enlargement of the prostate, unless otherwise directed by a doctor.
Halls Cough Suppressant Tablets	As directed on label.	Available in maximum-strength *(Halls Plus)*, as well as regular. Do not take for a persistent or chronic cough, or if you have excessive phlegm, unless otherwise directed by a doctor.

N'ICE Medicated Sugarless Throat & Cough Lozenges	As directed on label.	Soothing lozenges that come in 6 varieties. Adults and children over 6 can take up to 10 lozenges a day. Same warnings as *Halls Cough Suppressant Tablets.*
Robitussin-Pediatric Cough Suppressant	As directed on label.	No common side effects. Minor stomach discomfort, dizziness, and sleepiness occur only infrequently. Do not use if you are taking MAO inhibitors or for two weeks after you have stopped. Same warnings as *Halls Cough Suppressant Tablets.*
Sucrets 4-Hour Cough Suppressant Lozenges	As directed on label.	Do not use with MAO inhibitors. Do not exceed maximum of 6 lozenges every 24 hours; for adults and children over 6. Same warnings as *Halls Cough Suppressant Tablets.*
Vicks Cough Drops	As directed on label.	Available in extra strength, as well. Same warnings as *Halls Cough Suppressant Tablets.*
Nasal Congestion Medication		
4-Way Nasal Spray	As directed on label.	Available in *Fast-Acting* and *Long-Lasting* formulas. No common side effects. Nasal irritation or dryness occurs occasionally.
Afrin Nasal Spray	As directed on label.	No common side effects. Nasal irritation or dryness occurs occasionally.
Cheracol Nasal Spray Pump	As directed on label.	Same comments as *Afrin Nasal Spray.*

Neo-Synephrine Nasal Drops/ Sprays	As directed on label.	Available in a variety of strengths and formulas, including *Pediatric, Mild, Regular, Extra Strength,* and *Maximum Strength 12-Hour.* No common side effects. Dryness and irritation of the nasal passages occur only infrequently.
Pedicare Infants' Decongestant Drops	As directed on label.	No common side effects. Stomach discomfort, dizziness, and more severe adverse reactions occur only infrequently.
Vicks Sinex Nasal Spray	As directed on label.	Same comments as *Afrin Nasal Spray.*

When used responsibly, acetaminophen, aspirin, ibuprofen, ketoprofen, and naproxen sodium are safe and effective. Look for single-ingredient products. If you have questions or concerns regarding the safety and effectiveness of any product, consult your doctor or pharmacist.

Congestion, Nasal

See also Colds and Coughs; Flu; Sinusitis.

Nasal congestion is the partial blockage of the nasal passages due to inflammation of the mucous membranes that line them. There are a number of common causes for this condition: a cold or flu infection in the nasal passages; an allergic reaction; or an infection that has spread from the sinuses. Nasal congestion results in the spontaneous discharge of mucus from the nose.

Although similar, this condition is different from nasal obstruction, in which either one or both of the nasal passages are blocked to the extent that breathing is impaired. Inflammation may be involved in both nasal congestion and nasal obstruction, but the latter condition may also be caused by nasal polyps; injury that results in a hematoma (a collection of clotted blood); a deviated septum (the central partition in the nose); or a malignant tumor. Fortunately, malignant nasal tumors are quite rare. In children, nasal obstruction is frequently from enlarged adenoids. If nasal congestion persists, consult a physician.

OTC REMEDIES

There are a number of OTCs on the market for the relief of congestion. There is a variety of forms available to treat this congestion, among which are oral medication, nasal drops, and nasal sprays. Drops and sprays should be used as little as possible, because overuse can worsen the condition. Tablets and syrups are of less value and can cause drowsiness. Be sure to take necessary precautions. Always read the label carefully before using a product.

OTC Remedy	Dosage	Comments
4-Way Nasal Spray	As directed on label.	Available in *Fast-Acting* and *Long-Lasting* formulas. No common side effects. Nasal irritation and dryness occur only infrequently.
Actifed	As directed on label.	Combination decongestant and antihistamine, available in several formulas.

		Can cause drowsiness and dryness of the mucous membranes. Take necessary precautions and maintain fluid intake.
Afrin Nasal Spray	As directed on label.	No common side effects. Nasal irritation and dryness occur only infrequently.
Cheracol Nasal Spray Pump.	As directed on label.	Same comments as *Afrin Nasal Spray*.
Chlor-Trimeton Allergyl Decongestant Tablets	As directed on label.	Available in 4- and 12-hour formulas. Can cause drowsiness and dryness of the mucous membranes. Take necessary precautions and maintain fluid intake.
Neo-Synephrine Nasal Drops/ Sprays	As directed on label.	Available in a variety of strengths and formulas, including *Pediatric, Mild, Regular, Extra-Strength*, and *Maximum-Strength 12-Hour* formulas. No common side effects. Dryness and irritation of the nasal passages occur only infrequently.
PediaCare Infant's Decongestant Drops	As directed on label.	No common side effects. Stomach discomfort, dizziness, and more severe reactions occur only infrequently.
Vicks Sinex Decongestant Nasal Spray	As directed on label.	Also available in *12-Hour Formula*. Can cause headache and nasal passage irritation and dryness in some individuals.

If your congestion is a symptom of a cold, flu, allergy, or sinusitis, see the individual sections on those conditions for more information.

NATURAL REMEDIES

Diet is an important factor when it comes to dealing with congestion. Avoid mucus-forming foods, which include all dairy and cheese, eggs, wheat and oats, and starchy vegetables such as potatoes, yams, and squash. Raw foods are important, as is the elimination of salt. Drink lots of fluids, including water, herbal teas, broths, and juices, to cleanse the body and promote drainage.

Steam can also be very helpful for reducing congestion. Taking a hot shower or placing a towel-draped head over a bowl or sink filled with hot water may bring you relief. Keeping a humidifier running in the room will maintain moisture in the air. An added plus is that, if you are "mouth-breathing" as a result of the congestion, the extra moisture may prevent a very painful sore throat.

Constipation

No body function varies more from person to person and is more influenced by external factors than defecation. A wide range of bowel habits can be considered "normal." An individual knows his or her own body and feels discomfort when wastes are not properly excreted. Constipation is a condition involving the difficult or infrequent passage of feces. Sometimes this term is used to describe a feeling of incomplete evacuation or hardness of stool.

Age, diet, cultural patterns, and individual physiology influence bowel habits. In American society, healthy people have normal bowel movements anywhere from two to three times daily to two to three times weekly. Constipation is most commonly due to insufficient dietary fiber and fluids. Occasionally, constipation can result from drug therapy (for example, from antidepressants). It is also common during pregnancy.

Regular bowel movement is important to health. Without it, harmful toxins begin to form in the body. Constipation can cause other ailments, such as hemorrhoids, flatulence, insomnia, headaches, and indigestion. Therefore, it is important to resolve constipation problems.

OTC REMEDIES

The products listed in the following chart are *laxatives*—substances that stimulate the passage of feces. Be sure to use laxatives cautiously. Always read the label before using any product, and follow the instructions carefully.

OTC Remedy	Dosage	Comments
Cascara	As directed on label.	Stimulant laxative pills induce more rigorous smooth muscle action in the intestinal walls, to help expel the feces.

Docusate sodium *Correctol Extra Gentle Stool Softener*	As directed on label.	Increases liquid content of the stool, for easier passage.
Docusate sodium and phenolphthalein *Correctol Laxative Caplets/ Tablets; Ex-Lax Extra Gentle Laxative Pills; Feen-A-Mint Laxative Pills; Phillips' Laxative & Stool Softener Gelcaps*	As directed on label.	Stool softeners increase liquid content of the stool, for easier passage. Lubricants coat the fecal surface to facilitate excretion. Stimulant laxative pills induce more rigorous smooth muscle action in the intestinal walls, to help expel the feces.
Fiberall Powder	As directed on label.	Provides indigestible fiber that will increase the bulk of feces and promote lubrication and softening of stools.
Fibercon	As directed on label.	Same comments as *Fiberall Powder.*
Magnesium hydroxide *Phillips' Milk of Magnesia Laxatives*	As directed on label.	Causes surrounding tissues to release water into the bowels, making stools easier to pass and promoting bowel activity.
Metamucil	As directed on label.	Same comments as *Fiberall Powder.*
Phenolphthalein *Ex-Lax Laxative Tablets/Pills; Feen-A-Mint Laxative Gum*	As directed on label.	Stool softeners increase liquid content of the stool, for easier passage. Lubricants coat the fecal surface to facilitate excretion. Stimulant laxative pills induce more rigorous smooth muscle action in the intestinal walls, to help expel the feces.
Senna	As directed on label.	Same comments as *Cascara.*

If you have questions or concerns regarding the safety and effectiveness of any product, consult your doctor or pharmacist. Valid concerns have been expressed by authorities in the consumer-health field regarding the safety and effectiveness of certain chemicals. The following warning has been issued:

• Products that contain only magnesium hydroxide are considered safe for limited use only. Effective alternatives are products containing psyllium or castor oil.

NATURAL REMEDIES

A high-fiber diet rich in fruits and vegetables is a good alternative to laxative use if you are constipated. Prunes are a great natural laxative, as are psyllium products such as *Metamucil* and *Fibercon*. These are natural OTC products, and are listed in the "OTC Remedies" section. For other options, see the recommendations in the table below.

Keep in mind that the best natural approach to constipation is prevention. Add physical activity and exercise to your daily routine to speed the passage of waste material through your intestines. Drink six to eight glasses of water or fruit juice daily. Eat a diet high in brown rice, fresh fruits, and raw vegetables, especially the green leafy variety. If you suffer from occasional bouts of constipation, refrain from eating dairy products and foods made with white flour and/or sugar.

Natural Remedy	Dosage	Comments
Flaxseed oil	1 tbsp, daily	Take with food. Rich in essential fatty acids.
Psyllium	5 to 7 g, 1 to 2 times daily	A natural fiber.

Cuts and Scrapes

A cut or scrape involves damage to the skin and, sometimes, to the tissues and nerves underneath. We generally refer to a minor wound as a cut or scrape. Controlling the bleeding from a minor cut is usually the most immediate problem. The next most important thing to do is to prevent infection. A clean dressing will do the trick in most cases. Antiseptics are of limited value, but many people like to use them to be sure that the area is clean. If the injury is more serious than a minor cut, see a doctor or go to the emergency room for care.

OTC REMEDIES

The products listed in the following table provide relief from the pain and soreness of minor cuts and scrapes. Always read the label before using a product.

OTC Remedy	Application	Comments
Americaine Topical Anesthetic Spray and First Aid Ointment	Apply to wound, as directed on label.	Temporarily blocks the pain messages sent from the skin to the brain. Further skin irritation (including hives) due to use of this product is uncommon.

Bactine Antiseptic Anesthetic First Aid Liquid	Apply to wound, as directed on label.	Reduces inflammation, kills bacteria, and temporarily blocks pain messages sent from the skin to the brain. Further skin irritation due to use of this product is uncommon. Do not use if you are allergic to cortisone products.
Bactine First Aid Antibiotic Plus Anesthetic Ointment	Apply to wound, as directed on label.	Kills bacteria and temporarily blocks the pain messages sent from the skin to the brain. Further skin irritation due to use of this product is uncommon. Do not use if you are allergic to any of the following antibiotics or their related substances: chloramphenicol; gentamicin; mupirocin; neonycin; polymyxins. Overuse will lead to bacterial resistance.
BiCozene Creme	Apply to wound, as directed on label.	Topical anti-infective. Further skin irritation due to use of this product is uncommon.
Mycitracin Maximum Strength Triple Antibiotic First Aid Ointment	Apply to wound as directed on label.	Kills bacteria. Further skin irritation due to use of this product is uncommon. Do not use if you are allergic to any of the following antibiotics or their related substances: chloramphenicol; gentamicin; mupirocin; neomycin; polymyxins. Overuse will lead to bacterial resistance.

Mycitracin Plus Pain Reliever	Apply to wound, as directed on label.	Topical antibiotic. Further skin irritation due to use of this product is uncommon. Overuse will lead to bacterial resistance.
Neosporin Ointment	Apply to wound, as directed on label.	Also available in *Plus Maximum Strength*. Same comments as *Mycitracin Maximum Strength Triple Antibiotic First Aid Ointment*.

If you have questions or concerns regarding the safety and effectiveness of any product, consult your doctor or pharmacist. Valid concerns have been expressed by authorities in the consumer-health field regarding the safety and effectiveness of products that contain certain chemicals. The following warning has been issued:

- Do not use products containing only neomycin, polymyxin B, and bacitracin; or neomycin, polymyxin B, bacitracin, and hydrocortisone.

NATURAL REMEDIES

Aloe vera may be soothing to a cut or scrape. However, a topical natural remedy and a topical OTC treatment should not be used together. The OTC agents alone should work just fine. And in general, the body tends to heal itself when it comes to minor cuts and scrapes. Therefore, we do not strongly suggest a natural remedy for cuts and scrapes, other than keeping the area clean and protected.

Cystitis

This condition involves an infection of the urinary bladder and is caused by bacteria. Cystitis is very common among both men and women, but occurs more frequently in women. Approximately 85 percent of these infections are caused by *Escherichia coli,* a common form of intestinal bacteria. Another bacterium, *chlamydia,* may also cause this condition.

Often, cystitis occurs after sexual intercourse. Symptoms include: a burning sensation; an urgent desire to urinate; and frequent and even painful urination. Urine may appear cloudy and have a pungent, unpleasant odor. See your doctor for treatment, especially if blood appears in the urine.

OTC REMEDIES

The products listed in the following chart are analgesics—substances that relieve or reduce pain. If you have experienced side effects from any nonprescription pain relievers, do not take any of these remedies without consulting your doctor. Always read the label before using a product.

OTC Remedy	Dosage	Comments
Acetaminophen *Excedrin Aspirin-Free; Panadol; Tylenol*	325 mg regular strength; generally, 500 mg extra strength	Do not drink alcohol and use products containing acetaminophen. The combination can cause liver damage. Do not take with other analgesics. Some of these products, such as *Tylenol,* are available in regular, junior, and extra strength.

Aspirin (acetylsalicylic acid) *Ascriptin; Bayer; Bufferin; Ecotrin; Empirin; Excedrin Extra Strength*	325 mg regular strength; generally, 500 mg extra strength	If pregnant, consult your doctor before taking products containing aspirin. Do not take products containing aspirin during the last three months of pregnancy. Children and teens should not use products containing aspirin for colds, flus, or chickenpox. Do not take products containing aspirin if you have asthma, stomach problems, gastric ulcers, bleeding problems, or if you are allergic to aspirin.
Ibuprofen *Advil; Arthritis Foundation Ibuprofen; Motrin IB; Nuprin*	200 mg	If pregnant, consult your doctor before taking this remedy. Do not take products containing this ingredient during the last three months of pregnancy. Do not take this ingredient if you are allergic to aspirin. Do not take this ingredient with any other analgesics. Consult your doctor before taking this remedy with prescription drugs.
Ketoprofen *Orudis KT*	12.5 mg	Same comments as Ibuprofen.
Naproxen sodium *Aleve*	220 mg	If pregnant, consult your doctor before taking this remedy. Do not take products containing this ingredient during the last three months of pregnancy. Do not take this ingredient with any other analgesics. Consult your doctor before taking this remedy with prescription drugs.

When used responsibly, acetaminophen, aspirin, ibuprofen, ketoprofen, and naproxen sodium are safe and effective. Look for single-ingredient products. If you have questions or concerns regarding the safety and effectiveness of any product, consult your doctor or pharmacist.

NATURAL REMEDIES

To help speed the recovery process when you have a bladder infection, avoid citrus fruits, alcohol, products containing caffeine, carbonated beverages, and chocolate. Increase liquid intake—drink 8 ounces of water every hour. Consider adding pure cranberry juice to your diet, as well as the other supplements listed in the table below. Also, hot baths can be very soothing.

To help prevent bladder infections, urinate frequently. Wash and dry the genital and anal areas of the body regularly. Women who are prone to bladder infections should avoid using tampons and should switch to white cotton underwear.

Natural Remedy	Dosage	Comments
Cranberry *Cranactin*	As directed on label.	There is good evidence that cranberry extract can prevent bacterial adherence to the bladder wall, but *Cranactin* is one of the few products that have been tested for this activity.

Cranberry Juice	8 to 16 oz, daily	100-percent pure cranberry juice is preferred. Cranberry juice cocktail is more readily available, but may not be as effective and provides a significant number of calories due to its sugar content.
Multivitamin/ mineral*	See pages 14 to 20.	See pages 14 to 20.
Uva ursi	250 to 500 mg, 3 times daily	Choose a standardized product that contains 20-percent arbutin. Widely used in Europe for treating urinary tract infections.
Vitamin C*	500 mg, 3 times daily	Promotes bladder and kidney health.

* It is important that the discussed nutrients be part of a basic vitamin/mineral regimen so that the total daily amount of each nutrient obtained from both a multivitamin/mineral and other supplements is approximately the dosage indicated above.

Dandruff

Contrary to a number of television commercials, dandruff will not ruin your work or love life. However, it can be a nuisance and an embarrassment. Dandruff is an inflammatory scaling disease of the scalp, face, and sometimes other areas of the body. Its onset is gradual. The obvious signs are the scaly flakes of dandruff and the itching of the scalp or other affected areas. This condition is caused by a dysfunction of the sebaceous glands. Mild cases can be self-treated. Consult a dermatologist for advice on cleansing lotions or for treatment if the condition is severe.

OTC REMEDIES

The products listed in the following table are shampoos that are formulated to reduce dandruff problems. Always read the label before using a product.

OTC Remedy	Application	Comments
Head & Shoulders Intensive Treatment Dandruff Shampoo	As directed on bottle.	Reduces the rate of growth of cells on the scalp.
Selsun Blue Dandruff Shampoo	As directed on bottle.	Reduces the rate of growth of cells on the scalp.
Selsun Gold for Women	As directed on bottle.	Reduces the rate of growth of cells on the scalp.
Tegrin Dandruff Shampoo	As directed on bottle.	Reduces the rate of growth of cells on the scalp.

NATURAL REMEDIES

An experienced nutritionist may provide useful information about treating dandruff. A diet high in raw foods seems to help reduce this condition. Also, avoid fried foods, dairy products, sugar, flour, chocolate, nuts, and seafood, as these items seem to worsen dandruff. The Five-A-Day Diet (see page 21) is a good general guide. Finally, the table below offers some natural remedies.

Natural Remedy	Dosage	Comments
Flaxseed oil	1 tsp, daily	Helps to maintain balance of fatty acids, promoting healthy skin and scalp.
Multivitamin/ mineral	See pages 14 to 20.	See pages 14 to 20.

Dental Problems

See also Bruxism; Teething; Toothache.

Dental problems generally involve disorders of the teeth and gums. Many factors can contribute to dental problems, including: improper dental care; poor nutrition; excessive sugar and alcohol; smoking; certain drugs; and certain diseases. Tooth decay is one of the most common dental disorders. It is caused when bacteria in the mouth mix with remnants of food and the mouth's natural excretions, forming *plaque*. This sticky substance clings to the teeth and houses the bacteria, which continue to feed off sugars in foods. As these bacteria continue to thrive, they produce an acid that causes the teeth to lose calcium and phosphorus. This is why it is important to remove the plaque from teeth. If it remains and continues this process, the tooth decays in layers—first the enamel, then the dentin, and finally the pulp. In advanced stages, toothaches and even infections and abscesses occur.

In addition to tooth decay, improper dental care can result in *periodontal diseases* such as gingivitis and pyorrhea. ("Periodontal" indicates conditions that are near the tooth.) Gingivitis is an early stage of periodontal disease. It involves the swelling of the gum due to deposits of plaque caused primarily by food particles, bacteria, and mucus. If left untreated, infection and bleeding occur. Over time, gingivitis can develop into pyorrhea. At this stage, infections are caused by bacteria that get between the teeth and gums. These infections can become so severe that they attack the bone in the jaw and wear it away.

OTC REMEDIES

There are quite a few OTC treatments available that can reduce or alleviate the symptoms associated with some dental problems. The products listed in the first section of the following table are analgesics— substances that reduce or relieve pain. These analgesics also combat fever, which may occur during a dental infection. If you have experienced side effects from any nonprescription pain reliever, do not take any of these remedies without consulting your doctor. Also listed are topical pain relievers and helpful toothpastes. Always read the label before using a product.

OTC Remedy	Dosage	Comments
Oral Pain-Relieving Medications		
Acetaminophen *Excedrin Aspirin-Free; Panadol; Tylenol*	325 mg regular strength; generally, 500 mg extra strength	Do not drink alcohol and use products containing acetaminophen. The combination can cause liver damage. Do not take with other analgesics. Some of these products, such as *Tylenol,* are available in various strengths.
Aspirin (acetylsalicylic acid) *Ascriptin; Bayer; Bufferin; Ecotrin; Empirin; Excedrin Extra Strength*	325 mg regular strength; generally, 500 mg extra strength	If pregnant, consult your doctor before taking products containing aspirin. Do not take products containing aspirin during the last three months of pregnancy. Children and teens should not use products containing aspirin for colds, flus, or chickenpox.

		Do not take products containing aspirin if you have asthma, stomach problems, gastric ulcers, bleeding problems, or if you are allergic to aspirin.
Ibuprofen *Advil; Arthritis Foundation Ibuprofen; Motrin IB; Nuprin*	200 mg	If pregnant, consult your doctor before taking this remedy. Do not take products containing this ingredient during the last three months of pregnancy. Do not take this ingredient if you are allergic to aspirin. Do not take this ingredient with any other analgesics. Consult your doctor before taking this remedy with prescription drugs.
Ketoprofen *Orudis KT*	12.5 mg	Same comments as Ibuprofen.
Naproxen sodium *Aleve*	220 mg	If pregnant, consult your doctor before taking this remedy. Do not take products containing this ingredient during the last three months of pregnancy. Do not take this ingredient with any other analgesics. Consult your doctor before taking this remedy with prescription drugs.

Topical Medications

Anbesol	As directed on label.	Temporarily blocks the pain messages sent from the affected area to the brain. No common side effects. Increased irritation from use of this product is unusual. Keep in mind that proper treatment of the disorder is still necessary.

Orajel Maximum Strength Toothache Medicine	As directed on label.	Same comments as *Anbesol*.
Orajel Perioseptic	As directed on label.	Topical antiseptic (kills bacteria).

Toothpastes and Other Tooth-Care Products

Biotene Gum/ Mouthwash/ Toothpaste	As directed on package.	Contain a mild antibacterial and an enzyme that converts mouth sugars into hydrogen peroxide. Toothpaste and mouthwash are specifically helpful for dry mouth—a major undertreated condition.
Crest Sensitivity Protection Toothpaste (for Sensitive Teeth and Cavity Prevention)	As directed on tube.	Formulated to clean and protect especially vulnerable teeth and gums.
Dental Care by Arm & Hammer	As directed on tube.	Uses ingredients to decrease plaque.
Dental Gum by Breath Assure	As directed on package.	Uses ingredients to decrease plaque.
Sensodyne Toothpaste (for Sensitive Teeth and Cavity Prevention)	As directed on tube.	This product is available in several flavors, as well as with baking soda. Same comments as *Crest Sensitivity Protection Toothpaste*.

When used responsibly, acetaminophen, aspirin, ibuprofen, ketoprofen, and naproxen sodium are safe and effective. Look for single-ingredient products. If you have questions or concerns regarding the safety and effectiveness of any product, consult your doctor or pharmacist.

NATURAL REMEDIES

Once dental problems set in, they are best managed by a dental-care professional and the OTC products that have been prepared for oral disorders. Natural remedies are more applicable to the *prevention* of dental problems. Dental health involves a commitment to daily tooth and gum care. This includes brushing and flossing, stimulating the gums with wooden toothpicks, and using a plaque-fighting dental rinse. Change toothbrushes every month. For the treatment of gum disease, brush teeth with a very soft toothbrush.

In addition to maintaining proper dental hygiene, avoid sugar, sweets, soft drinks, and refined foods. To enhance your general health, which will in turn enhance your dental health, follow the well-known Five-A-Day Diet (see page 21) or another diet recommended by a trained nutritionist. Proper supplementation may also help to maintain dental health. See the table below for suggestions.

Natural Remedy	Dosage	Comments
Ginkgo biloba *Bioginkgo; Ginkogin; Ginkai; Ginkgomax; Ginkoba; Ginkgo Go*	*Generic products:* 80 mg, 2 times daily; *Brand name products:* As directed on label.	Effect on blood platelets may help to maintain healthy gums. Some people experience a slight headache during the first few days of use, but this side effect usually subsides within the first week.

Multivitamin/	See pages 14 to 20.	See pages 14 to 20.
mineral,		
including		
antioxidants		

Depression

See Mood Disorders.

Dermatitis

See also Skin Problems.

Dermatitis is characterized by redness, swelling, crusting, scaling, and itching of the skin. For this book's purposes, dermatitis and eczema are considered the same condition. (Medical experts disagree on how to distinguish between Eczematous dermatitis and eczema.) Dermatitis can be caused by a sensitivity to a chemical, a food allergy, an overabundance of yeast, or a lack of necessary fatty acids or zinc in the body. Emotional factors may also contribute to this condition.

Contact dermatitis may be acute or chronic. It is caused by irritating substances that come into contact with the skin. The affected area is clearly defined. Chemical irritants in soaps, detergents, and similar products may cause this condition to develop over a few days. Stronger chemicals—those in industrial products, for example—may cause this condition to erupt in only minutes.

Allergic contact dermatitis is a delayed reaction that appears anywhere from six to ten days after exposure to the allergen. The rash resulting from contact with poison ivy is an example. Topical drugs, antibiotics, antihistamines, anesthetics, and antiseptic products can cause this condition in some people. Sometimes allergic contact dermatitis can even take years to develop.

Atopic dermatitis is a chronic itching and superficial inflammation of the skin. In fact, itching is a constant aspect of atopic dermatitis. There is often a personal and/or family history of related problems associated with this condition, such as asthma or hay fever. Airborne allergens, emotional stress, chemical irritants, prescription or OTC drugs, changes in temperature or humidity, bacterial skin infections, and wool garments can aggravate this condition.

Seborrheic dermatitis, also known as seborrhea, is an inflammatory scaling disease of the scalp, face, chest, and possibly other areas of the body. This condition appears gradually, and dandruff is an early sign. Seborrhea is characterized by oily skin. It is probably best not to use ointments to treat it. Cleansing lotions with a drying agent are usually preferred.

Do not self-diagnose any of these conditions. See a physician if you suspect that you have dermatitis. He or she will give you a treatment plan that may include OTCs and natural remedies. If so, you can self-manage this condition.

OTC REMEDIES

The products listed in the following table are topical medications that offer relief from the symptoms of dermatitis. Always read the label before using a product.

OTC Remedy	Application	Comments
Caldecort Anti-Itch Cream/Spray	As directed on label.	Available in *Light Cream,* as well. Reduces inflammation. Further skin irritation due to use of this product is uncommon. Do not use if you are allergic to any cortisone products.
Cortaid Cream/ Ointment/ Spray	As directed on label.	The regular- and maximum-strength formulas are available in cream and ointment forms, while the maximum-strength formula is also available in spray form. Reduces inflammation. Further skin irritation due to use of this product is uncommon. Do not use if you are allergic to any cortisone products.
Cortizone-5 Creme/Ointment	As directed on label.	Reduces inflammation. Further skin irritation due to use of the product is uncommon. Do not use if you are allergic to any cortisone products.
Cortizone-10 Creme/Ointment	As directed on label.	Same comments as *Cortizone-5 Creme/Ointment.*
Cortizone for Kids Anti-Itch Creme	As directed on label.	Same comments as *Cortizone-5 Creme/Ointment.*

Eucerin Creme	As directed on label.	Moisturizes dry and irritated skin. Discontinue use if irritation occurs.

NATURAL REMEDIES

To help alleviate dermatitis, drink lots of water. In addition, follow a healthy diet, such as the Five-A-Day Diet (see page 21) or another diet recommended by a trained nutritionist. Some people who suffer from dermatitis have found that omitting wheat, rye, oats, and barley from the diet for six weeks alleviates the condition.

Alternative/complementary practitioners may offer effective care if conventional advice is not resolving the problem. Also, the following table lists some natural substances that may improve the condition of affected skin.

Natural Remedy	Dosage	Comments
Flaxseed oil	Up to 1 tbsp (or 1 to 3 tsp), daily	Helps to maintain proper fatty acid balance, promoting healthy skin.
Multivitamin/ mineral,* including anti-oxidants	See pages 14 to 20.	See pages 14 to 20.
Zinc*	30 mg, daily	Take with a meal. Doses in excess of 100 mg can depress immune function. If your multivitamin/mineral already contains this amount of zinc, there is no need for further supplementation.

* It is important that the discussed nutrients be part of a basic vitamin/mineral regimen so that the total daily amount of each nutrient obtained from both a multivitamin/mineral and other supplements is approximately the dosage indicated above.

Diaper Rash

This common condition is usually caused by the reaction of the skin to the powerful enzymes and chemicals in feces and urine. Diapers can trap these irritants against the skin, resulting in inflammation. Diaper rash can be caused by soaps, disposable diapers, plastic pants, and/or diarrhea. With this condition, the skin will be sore, tender, and red. Keep in mind that diet and nutrition may also play a role in the appearance and severity of diaper rash.

Diaper rash is especially common in infants around nine months of age. Watch for any of the following signs that the condition is worsening: changes in the severity of the rash; fluid discharge from the irritated area; swelling; fever; increased redness; increased irritability in the baby. If the child shows any of these symptoms, contact a doctor. In cases in which the baby's skin is smooth, shiny, and bright red, the rash may be caused by a fungus called *candida albicans*. This fungus is common among women and men, and can be easily transmitted to a baby. A doctor or nurse should diagnose the cause of the baby's rash.

OTC REMEDIES

The products listed in the following chart help to relieve the symptoms of diaper rash. Always read the label before using any product.

Do not use these products on broken skin. They are for external use only; if ingested, call the Poison

Control Center. If no improvement is seen after seven days, consult with a physician.

OTC Remedy	Application	Comments
A and D Medicated Diaper Rash Ointment	As directed on label.	Original *A and D Ointment* may also be of help. Kills fungus cells.
Caldesene Medicated Ointment/ Powder	As directed on label.	Kills fungus cells. Powder absorbs excess moisture from affected area. Keep powder away from child's face to avoid inhalation.
Clocream Skin Protectant	As directed on label.	Provides protective coating and and maintains a clean environment for the skin.
Daily Care from Desitin Diaper Rash Prevention Ointment	As directed on label.	Same comments as *Clocream Skin Protectant*.
Desitin Cornstarch Baby Powder (with Zinc Oxide)	As directed on label.	Absorbs excess moisture and promotes healing. Keep powder away from child's face to avoid inhalation.

NATURAL REMEDIES

The use of cotton diapers instead of disposable diapers can reduce diaper rash, as can changing diapers frequently. Whenever possible, allow the child to wear no diaper, as this will permit healthy air circulation. Sunlight is also helpful. (Avoid sunburn.) A baking-soda rinse for the area can greatly contribute to healing the rash. Finally, if OTCs are ineffective, try steeping 2 tablespoons of dried chamomile in 2 cups of boiling water for ten minutes. Cool the mixture to room temperature (test it on your wrist). Then, dip a soft washcloth into the liquid and apply it to the rash as often as possible.

Diarrhea

Diarrhea is characterized by increased fluidity, frequency, and volume of fecal discharge. Common symptoms include runny stools, cramps, thirst, abdominal pain, and fever. Vomiting may sometimes accompany diarrhea, as well. This condition can be attributed to a number of different causes, such as: food poisoning; bacteria and viruses; stress; incomplete digestion; certain drugs; and drinking water in other countries (traveler's diarrhea).

Diarrhea itself is a symptom; the underlying disorder must be identified and treated. If you have diarrhea, do not take corrective medications for the first day or two, as diarrhea is an effective way for the body to rid itself of toxins. Severe diarrhea requires a doctor's attention. Symptomatic treatment may be necessary while medical evaluation is undertaken, because there can be serious consequences as a result of this condition.

OTC REMEDIES

The products listed in the following table are formulated to correct the problem of diarrhea. Always read the label before using a product.

OTC Remedy	Dosage	Comments
Attapulgite *Kaopectate Liquid/Maximum Strength Caplets*	As directed on label.	Reduces water loss, while absorbing toxins and harmful bacteria. No common side effects. Mild constipation due to use of this product occurs only infrequently.
Bismuth subsalicylate *Pepto-Bismol Original Liquid/ Caplets/Tablets*	As directed on label.	Absorbs some bacteria; induces the intestinal wall to absorb fluids and electrolytes; reduces inflammation and overactivity of intestinal muscles and wall. Commonly results in very dark stools and a darkened tongue. These side effects are not harmful.
Loperamide hydrochloride *Immodium A-D; Kaopectate 1-D Caplets; Maalox Anti-Diarrheal Caplets*	As directed on label.	Disrupts nerve action in digestive tract, reducing intestinal activity. No common side effects.

If you have questions or concerns regarding the safety and effectiveness of any product, consult your doctor or pharmacist. Valid concerns have been expressed by authorities in the consumer-health field regarding the safety and effectiveness of the chemical loperamide. The following warning has been issued:

• Products containing only loperamide should be taken for limited use only.

NATURAL REMEDIES

To restore your bowels to normal function, increase your potassium intake. Food and drink are the best sources of potassium. For example, one banana supplies ten times the amount of potassium as a 99-milligram daily supplement dose. In fact, you cannot get the amount of potassium you need from supplements alone. Another option is to drink plenty of potassium-rich fluids, such as *Pedialyte* or *Gatorade*.

Restructuring your diet will contribute to digestive health. When trying to remedy diarrhea, stay away from white sugar and refined carbohydrates. Also avoid the following foods and substances which may worsen diarrhea: dairy products; fruit juices; soft drinks; grapes; figs; dates; honey; "sugar-free" gum and mints; antacids; and caffeine-containing products, including coffee, tea, sodas, and some OTC headache remedies.

Rice water, taken three times daily, can help treat diarrhea effectively. After the condition improves, eating rice will assist in maintaining normalized bowel movements. Also, yogurt, rolled oats, and vegetables that are steamed or in soups can help.

If chronic stress is contributing to or causing your diarrheal condition, use stress-management techniques. Examples are: yoga; meditation; a regular exercise program; and massage therapy. And if your diarrhea is due to an infection, be sure to get plenty of rest so that your immune system can restore itself.

To avoid dehydration from diarrhea, drink plenty of liquids—water, vegetable and fruit (diluted and unsweetened) juices, and broths. The loss of too much fluid from the body disrupts bacteria and electrolyte balance. For children, this balance can easily be restored through such foods as applesauce and yogurt. It is important to note that too much vitamin C and too much magnesium can also cause diarrhea in some people. Finally, the remedies listed in the following table may further help relieve the symptoms of this condition.

Natural Remedy	Dosage	Comments
To Restore Balance to the Bowel		
Acidophilus capsules/tablets/liquid/powder *(Lactobacillus acidophilus)*	As directed on label.	Helps restore friendly bacteria in the gut. While acidophilus, alone, is helpful, you can also find products that contain additional friendly bacteria. Only purchase products that have been refrigerated, to ensure and maintain activity.
For Cramps/Abdominal Pain		
Ginger extract	2 capsules, 4 times daily	Standardized extract is preferred, but if it is not available, you can use ginger root capsules. There is no established effective amount for the root capsules. You might try 4 capsules, 4 times daily, and adjust as needed.

Dry Skin

See Skin Problems.

Ear Infections

Infection of the external ear is the most common source of earache. (During such infections, the middle ear may also be involved.) This condition affects about 95 percent of children. Persistent infection can lead to serious damage of the eardrum. Loss of hearing is a possibility in some cases. When the outer ear is infected, the ear canal becomes inflamed from the outside to the eardrum. Pain, fluid discharge, low-grade fever, sensitivity of the ear to touch, and temporary loss of hearing may occur. See a doctor immediately if there is sudden pain, bleeding, blood in the fluid discharge, ringing in the ears, and/or dizziness.

Middle-ear infections are also common in infants and children. This condition is usually caused by infection that is located behind the eardrum. Fever, pressure, a sense of fullness, and earache are common symptoms. High altitudes, cold weather, unsanitary conditions, and air travel can all lead to infection of the ear. If you have an earache, do not blow your nose; doing so may damage your ear.

Most ear infections occur in children and can result in serious problems. It is therefore essential to see a doctor as soon as possible. Antibiotics may be necessary. Once the severity of the infection has been evaluated and your physician has provided guidance, you can manage the pain with a number of OTC products and natural remedies.

OTC REMEDIES

The products listed in the following table are analgesics—substances that relieve or reduce pain. They also combat fever. If you have experienced side effects from any nonprescription pain relievers, do not take any of these remedies without consulting your doctor. Always read the label before using a product.

OTC Remedy	Dosage	Comments
Acetaminophen *Excedrin Aspirin-Free; Panadol; Tylenol*	325 mg regular strength; generally, 500 mg extra strength	Do not drink alcohol and use products containing acetaminophen. The combination can cause liver damage. Do not take with other analgesics. Some of these products, such as *Tylenol,* are available in regular, junior, and extra strength.
Aspirin (acetylsalicylic acid) *Ascriptin; Bayer; Bufferin; Ecotrin; Empirin; Excedrin Extra Strength*	325 mg regular strength; generally, 500 mg extra strength	If pregnant, consult your doctor before taking products containing aspirin. Do not take products containing aspirin during the last three months of pregnancy. Children and teens should not use products containing aspirin for colds, flus, or chickenpox. Do not take products containing aspirin if you have asthma, stomach problems, gastric ulcers, bleeding problems, or if you are allergic to aspirin.
Ibuprofen *Advil; Arthritis Foundation Ibuprofen; Motrin IB; Nuprin*	200 mg	If pregnant, consult your doctor before taking this remedy. Do not take products containing this ingredient during the last three months of pregnancy. Do not take this ingredient if

		you are allergic to aspirin. Do not take this ingredient with any other analgesics. Consult your doctor before taking this remedy with prescription drugs.
Ketoprofen *Orudis KT*	12.5 mg	Same comments as Ibuprofen.
Naproxen Sodium *Aleve*	220 mg	If pregnant, consult your doctor before taking this remedy. Do not take products containing this ingredient during the last three months of pregnancy. Do not take this ingredient with any other analgesics. Consult your doctor before taking this remedy with prescription drugs.

When used responsibly, acetaminophen, aspirin, ibuprofen, ketoprofen, and naproxen sodium are safe and effective. Look for single-ingredient products. If you have questions or concerns regarding the safety and effectiveness of any product, consult your doctor or pharmacist.

NATURAL REMEDIES

To alleviate an earache, fill a dropper bottle with olive oil. Hold the bottle under hot running water until the oil is warm when applied to the wrist. Then fill the ear canal with the oil and cover it with a cotton plug. This should be done three or four times throughout the day. Also, a heating pad, hot water bottle, or warm washcloth placed around the ear—especially in front, behind, and below—should provide relief.

Ear infections can be caused by food allergies. Common food items that cause such allergic reactions are: milk and other dairy products; eggs; wheat; corn; peanuts; and citrus fruits. If you suffer from food allergies, white sugar and refined carbohydrates in the diet should be decreased. Whole foods should be added to the diet, as well as garlic and onions for their infection-fighting, immune-enhancing effects.

Be careful not to get water in the ear—from swimming, showers, etc.—while you have an infection. It is important to keep the ear dry. Keeping a cotton plug in the ear at all times will maintain dryness and warmth.

Eczema

See Dermatitis.

Eye Problems

Pain in the eye is a critical symptom. If it is not caused by something immediately identifiable, such as a particle in the eye, the common cold, a sinus infection, or an injury, eye problems should be investigated right away. They may be a sign of another physical disease. For example, protruding eyes may signal a thyroid problem; yellow eyes may indicate jaundice from hepatitis or gall bladder disease; and blurred vision may be a result of diabetes or hypertension. There are also many serious disorders specifically afflicting the eye, such as conjunctivitis, glaucoma, and cataracts. These conditions require a doctor's attention. Except when you "get something in your eye" momentarily, or experience redness and discomfort from environmental allergens, do not self-diagnose and treat eye problems. But during those times when it is just a minor irritation, there are products and natural remedies that can ease your discomfort. Common symptoms of simple irritation include bloodshot eyes, watery eyes, and stinging/burning.

Straining, sneezing, or coughing can cause hemorrhaging in the eyes. Usually, this looks far worse than it is. The redness will disappear within two weeks, as the blood is absorbed. Drugs are of no help with this common occurrence. Patience is the only remedy.

It is important to note that some prescription drugs may cause eye problems. For example, corticosteroids, diuretics, and some antibiotics have been known to negatively affect the eyes. Even aspirin can cause problems on occasion. Be sure that you are familiar with possible side effects before taking prescription medications.

OTC REMEDIES

The following table lists several products that can reduce or relieve the symptoms of such minor conditions as bloodshot eyes, eyestrain, or watery eyes. Always read the label before using a product. If you have had an allergic reaction to any decongestant eye-care solutions in the past, do not use these products.

OTC Remedy	Application	Comments
Clear Eyes ACR Astringent Eye Drops	As directed on label.	Constricts blood vessels in the eyes to relieve redness. If further eye irritation occurs, discontinue use and call a doctor.
Clear Eyes Lubricant Eye Drops	As directed on label.	Relieves dryness. If further eye irritation occurs, discontinue use and call a doctor.
Clear Eyes Redness Reliever Eye Drops	As directed on label.	Constricts the blood vessels in the eyes to relieve redness. If further eye irritation occurs, discontinue use and call a doctor.
Lavoptik Eye Wash	As directed on label.	Gently rinses the eye. If further eye irritation occurs, discontinue use and call a doctor.
Murine Lubricant Eye Drops	As directed on label.	Relieves dryness. If further eye irritation occurs, discontinue use and call a doctor.
Murine Lubricant Plus Redness Reliever Eye Drops	As directed on label.	The lubricant relieves dryness, while the redness reliever constricts the small blood vessels in the eyes. If further eye irritation occurs, discontinue use and call a doctor.
Visine Maximum Strength Allergy Relief Eye Drops	As directed on label.	Topical antiseptic with boric acid as main ingredient. If further eye irritation occurs, discontinue use and call a doctor.

Visine *Redness* *Reliever* *Eye Drops*	As directed on label.	Available in *Maximum Strength, Moisturizing,* and *Original* formulas. The moisturizing formula provides a lubricant to relieve dryness, while the redness reliever constricts the small blood vessels in the eyes. If further eye irritation occurs, discontinue use and call a doctor.

Keep in mind that overindulgence with alcohol can cause bloodshot eyes. Consider cutting back on alcohol intake rather than using eyewashes to cover up the telltale redness in the eyes.

NATURAL REMEDIES

The products listed in the following table are helpful in maintaining healthy eye functioning and for the prevention of eye degeneration, but should not be used for treating any eye *condition* unless prescribed by a physician.

Natural Remedy	Application	Comments
Bilberry *Bilberry 20-20; Ocumax 20-20*	240 to 480 mg, daily	Use standardized extract that provides 25-percent anthocyanosides. An antioxidant that may prevent formation of cataracts and improve circulation to the eyes.
Grape-seed extract or **Pine bark extract** *Pycnogenol*	50 to 100 mg, daily	Rich source of antioxidants that can prevent premature aging of the eyes. Grape-seed extract and pine bark extract are comparable substances.

Fatigue

See also Chronic Fatigue Syndrome.

Fatigue is a symptom, not a disorder. Poor diet and emotional stress are two major causes of this condition. Lack of physical exercise also contributes to fatigue. Alcohol, cigarette smoking, caffeine, and certain drugs deplete the body of energy, as well. Furthermore, a lack of mental or intellectual stimulation, and the absence of joy in life, can lead to fatigue. Some serious illnesses can cause this condition: allergies; anemia; anxiety; cancer; candidiasis; circulatory problems; depression; diabetes; Epstein-Barr virus; and mononucleosis.

If you have been suffering from chronic or long-term fatigue, see your doctor to find out whether you suffer from chronic fatigue syndrome or another condition. If the doctor rules out medical conditions as the cause of fatigue, then there are some remedies that may help.

OTC REMEDIES

Short-term use of caffeine products are helpful on occasion for most adults, and have few side effects. In an urgent situation, such as driving a vehicle while fatigued, we suggest *No Doze*, an OTC that supplies 200 milligrams of caffeine. However, this and other stimulant products should be used only when absolutely necessary. In the long term, caffeine stimulants actually worsen fatigue, as they place excess stress on the body. Therefore, it is best not to rely on OTC products for the resolution of fatigue. Instead, make healthy lifestyle changes.

NATURAL REMEDIES

Healthy lifestyle habits are key in the fight against fatigue. Include lots of fresh fruits and vegetables, grains, seeds, and nuts in your diet, all of which will provide you with good nutrition and more energy. Try following the Five-A-Day Diet (see page 21) or another diet recommended by a trained nutritionist.

Stress-management and relaxation techniques such as yoga and meditation are helpful, as they ultimately increase energy. It is also very important to get the proper amount of sleep each night—for most people, this means six to eight hours of solid rest—so that your body can get accustomed to a healthy pattern. See a health-care professional if you find that emotional problems are keeping you from healthy lifestyle habits.

Avoid dependence on caffeine. While it gives a temporary boost to the central nervous system, it stresses other bodily systems. Excessive caffeine will actually result in fatigue. Also avoid alcohol, sugar, white flour products, and high-fat and processed foods.

The following table lists several natural substances that allow your body to feel more invigorated. As part of a balanced diet, they may be very beneficial.

Natural Remedy	Dosage	Comments
CoQ$_{10}$ (coenzyme Q$_{10}$, also called ubiquinone)	75 mg, daily	Helps the body to produce energy at the cellular level. This substance is most recognized for its cardiovascular benefits.
Multivitamin/ mineral, including antioxidants	See pages 14 to 20.	See pages 14 to 20.
NADH *ENADA*	10 mg daily	A stable form of the nutrient NADH that has been shown to alleviate some symptoms associated with CFS.
Siberian ginseng *(Eleutherococcus senticosus)*	*Standardized Extract:* 200 mg, daily; *Dried root:* 2,000 to 4,000 mg, daily	Standardized extract is preferable to the dried root. If you choose the extract, purchase extract that contains at least 1-percent Eleutheroside E. Enhances energy and well-being. Do not use this herb if you suffer from any of the following: heart disorder; high blood pressure; hypoglycemia.

Fever

The presence of fever indicates that something is wrong. Fever is a symptom of an underlying disorder that must be identified and treated. The body's normal temperature is between 98°F and 99°F. A higher temperature is actually part of the body's defense system; it is an attempt to destroy invading bacteria, viruses, and/or other microorganisms. If a fever is under 102°F in an adult, or under 103°F in a child, there is no serious cause for concern. In fact, it is beneficial to let the fever run its natural course as part of the body's self-healing process. However, if the fever goes above those temperatures or lasts for more than a day, consult a doctor immediately. Once the cause of the fever has been identified and any necessary treatment is provided, there are products that you can take or natural remedies that you can follow to reduce the fever.

Rising fever is usually a sign that the condition is worsening. A fever that is too high, or a fever that lasts for a long period of time, can cause dehydration and brain damage. It is important to drink plenty of water or juices when a fever is present. Never give aspirin to a child with a fever. If the child is suffering from a strain of the flu or from chickenpox, the aspirin could cause Reye's syndrome, a serious and sometimes fatal neurological disorder.

OTC REMEDIES

The products listed in the following chart are analgesics—substances that relieve or reduce pain—that also combat fever. If you have experienced side effects from any nonprescription pain relievers, do not take any of these remedies without consulting your doctor. Always read the label before using a product.

OTC Remedy	Dosage	Comments
Acetaminophen *Excedrin Aspirin-Free; Panadol; Tylenol*	325 mg regular strength; generally, 500 mg extra strength	Do not drink alcohol and use products containing acetaminophen. The combination can cause liver damage. Do not take with other analgesics.

		Some products, such as *Tylenol*, are available in regular, junior, and extra strength.
Aspirin (acetylsalicylic acid) *Ascriptin; Bayer; Bufferin; Ecotrin; Empirin; Excedrin Extra Strength*	325 mg regular strength; generally, 500 mg extra strength	If pregnant, consult your doctor before taking products containing aspirin. Do not take products containing aspirin during the last three months of pregnancy. Children and teens should not use products containing aspirin for colds, flus, or chickenpox. Do not take products containing aspirin if you have asthma, stomach problems, gastric ulcers, bleeding problems, or if you are allergic to aspirin.
Ibuprofen *Advil; Arthritis Foundation Ibuprofen; Motrin IB; Nuprin*	200 mg	If pregnant, consult your doctor before taking this remedy. Do not take products containing this ingredient during the last three months of pregnancy. Do not take this ingredient if you are allergic to aspirin. Do not take this ingredient with any other analgesics. Consult your doctor before taking this remedy with prescription drugs.
Ketoprofen *Orudis KT*	12.5 mg	Same comments as Ibuprofen.
Naproxen sodium *Aleve*	220 mg	If pregnant, consult your doctor before taking this remedy. Do not take products containing this ingredient during the last three months of pregnancy. Do not take this ingredient with any other analgesics. Consult your doctor before taking this remedy with prescription drugs.

When used responsibly, acetaminophen, aspirin, ibuprofen, ketoprofen, and naproxen sodium are safe and effective. Look for single-ingredient products. If you have questions or concerns regarding the safety and effectiveness of any product, consult your doctor or pharmacist.

NATURAL REMEDIES

Drinking plenty of water and juices will keep you hydrated during the fever and will assist in flushing toxins out of your body. Cool baths help to reduce increased temperature. Be sure to get a lot of rest.

Flu (Influenza)

The flu, or influenza, is caused by highly contagious viruses that easily spread from person to person through coughing and sneezing. The respiratory tract is the main site of infection. The viruses mutate and, therefore, vaccination is of limited value. "Flu season" is an annual event, bringing much discomfort and suffering with it. Each year, many thousands of Americans die from influenza in conjunction with other conditions. But for most of us, a flu is treatable.

Usually, about three days after infection, the flu appears suddenly. At first, the symptoms are similar to those of the common cold—headaches, congestion, etc.—plus muscle aches and pains throughout the body. Later, a high fever may alternate with chills. A cough and dry throat is common, as is nausea and vomiting. Fatigue is so great that the flu sufferer has no appetite and cannot do anything but stay in bed. Rest and fluids are necessary. If the condition worsens, if it persists for longer than a week, or if the fever becomes higher than 102°F in adults and 103°F in children, consult a physician.

Keep in mind that sometimes products that lower fever interfere with the body's ability to heal itself. If it is not too high, allow the fever to run its course, as an elevated temperature is an effective immune response. However, do not let a dangerously high fever continue. Dehydration and damage to the brain can occur.

OTC REMEDIES

The products listed in the following table may bring relief from the symptoms of the flu. Those included in the first section are analgesics—substances that relieve or reduce pain and fever. If you have experienced side effects from any nonprescription pain relievers, do not take any of these remedies without consulting your doctor. Always read the label before using a product.

OTC Remedy	Dosage	Comments
For Pain, Fever, and General Flu Symptoms		
Acetaminophen *Children's Tylenol Cold Multi-Symptom Chewable Tablets/ Liquid; Children's Tylenol Cold Plus Cough Multi-Symptom*	Follow manufacturers' dosages.	Do not drink alcohol and use products containing acetaminophen. The combination can cause liver damage. Do not take with other analgesics. Some of these products, such as *Tylenol,* are available in regular, junior,

Chewable Tablets/ Liquid; Contac Severe Cold & Flu Non-Drowsy Caplets; Coricidin "D" Tablets; Drixoral Cold & Flu; Excedrin Aspirin-Free; Panadol; Theraflu Flu, Cold & Cough Medicine; Tylenol; Tylenol Cold Medicine Multi-Symptom Formula Tablets/Caplets

and extra strength. Also, *Theraflu* is available in regular and maximum strengths, as well as in nighttime and non-drowsy formulas.

Aspirin (acetylsalicylic acid) *Alka-Seltzer Plus Cold Medicine; Alka-Seltzer Plus Cold & Cough Medicine; Ascriptin; Bayer; Bufferin; Ecotrin; Empirin; Excedrin Extra Strength*	Follow manufacturers' dosages.	If pregnant, consult your doctor before taking products containing aspirin. Do not take products containing aspirin during the last three months of pregnancy. Children and teens should not use products containing aspirin for colds, flus, or chickenpox. Do not take products containing aspirin if you have asthma, stomach problems, gastric ulcers, bleeding problems, or if you are allergic to aspirin.
Ibuprofen *Advil; Advil Cold & Sinus; Arthritis Foundation Ibuprofen; Motrin IB; Motrin IB & Sinus; Nuprin*	200 mg	If pregnant, consult your doctor before taking this remedy. Do not take products containing this ingredient during the last three months of pregnancy. Do not take this ingredient if you are allergic to aspirin.

		Do not take this ingredient with any other analgesics. Consult your doctor before taking this remedy with prescription drugs.
Ketoprofen *Orudis KT*	12.5 mg	Same comments as Ibuprofen.
Naproxen sodium *Aleve*	220 mg	If pregnant, consult your doctor before taking this remedy. Do not take products containing this ingredient during the last three months of pregnancy. Do not take this ingredient with any other analgesics. Consult your doctor before taking this remedy with prescription drugs.

For Nasal Congestion

4-Way *Nasal Spray*	As directed on label.	Available in *Fast-Acting* and *Long-Lasting* formulas. No common side effects. Irritation or dryness of the nasal passages sometimes occurs.
Afrin Nasal Spray	As directed on label.	No common side effects. Irritation or dryness of the nasal passages sometimes occurs.
Cheracol Nasal Spray Pump	As directed on label.	Same comments as *Afrin Nasal Spray*.
Neo-Synephrine Nasal Drops/Sprays	As directed on label.	Available in a variety of strengths and formulas, including *Pediatric, Mild, Regular, Extra-Strength,* and *Maximum-Strength 12-Hour* formulas. Same comments as *Afrin Nasal Spray*.

Pediacare Infant's Decongestant Drops	As directed on label.	No common side effects. Stomach discomfort, dizziness, and more severe reactions occur only infrequently.
Vicks Sinex Nasal Spray	As directed on label.	Also available in *12-Hour Decongestant* spray. Same comments as *Afrin Nasal Spray*.

When used responsibly, acetaminophen, aspirin, ibuprofen, ketoprofen, and naproxen sodium are safe and effective. Look for single-ingredient products. If you have questions or concerns regarding the safety and effectiveness of any product, consult your doctor or pharmacist.

NATURAL REMEDIES

The best way to avoid the discomfort of the flu is to practice prevention. Make sure that your immune system is adequately stimulated to fight off disease. Healthy lifestyle habits are the key to this tactic. Eat a healthy diet, such as the Five-A-Day Diet (see page 21). Proper nutrition is paramount to health. Also, maintain a good multivitamin/mineral regimen, get adequate rest, and perform regular exercise. These lifestyle factors will keep your immunity functioning well. Finally, make a commitment to stress reduction through such programs as yoga and meditation.

If you do come down with the flu, be sure to drink lots of fluids and to get plenty of rest. The products listed in the following table will help to speed your recovery.

Natural Remedy	Dosage	Comments
Echinacea	300 mg, 3 times daily for 10 days	Purchase standardized extract tablets/capsules. Appears to lose its effectiveness over time. Therefore, this herb works best if taken for short periods of treatment. Do not use to treat immune-deficiency diseases.
Garlic	1 clove, daily, or the equivalent in caplets/tablets	Make sure the product you select states "Allicin Potential." This phrase indicates potency. Use as part of a maintenance regimen, not only to improve immune function, but to decrease the risk of heart disease and cancer, as well
Multivitamin/ mineral*	See pages 14 to 20.	See pages 14 to 20.
Vitamin C*	*First two days:* 1,000 mg, 4 times daily; *Following two days:* 1,000 mg, 2 times daily; *For maintenance:* 500 mg, 2 times daily	Works best if taken at the first sign of cold or flu. Safe for long-term maintenance.
Zinc lozenges	*First day:* dissolve 1 lozenge under the tongue every 2 hours; *Second day:* dissolve 1 lozenge under the tongue every 4 hours; *Next four days:* dissolve 1 tablet under the tongue every 6 hours	To be effective, use at the first sign of the flu. Some individuals experience mouth irritation with frequent use of zinc lozenges. If you do, experiment with different brands until you find the one that best suits you.

* It is important that the discussed nutrients be part of a basic vitamin/mineral regimen so that the total daily amount of each nutrient obtained from both a multivitamin/mineral and other supplements is approximately the dosage indicated above.

Food Allergy

A food allergy is quite simply an allergic reaction to a specific food. (This is not the same condition as a food intolerance, in which an individual cannot properly digest certain foods and experiences nausea, bloating, gas, etc., as a result.) Food allergies provoke the same symptoms as other allergies: skin rashes, possibly accompanied by gastrointestinal problems; congestion; mild asthma attacks. Common foods to induce allergic attacks include nuts, shellfish, soybeans, milk, eggs, chocolate, and wheat.

Some individuals react violently to food allergies. Even a tiny amount of the food can cause life-threatening symptoms. A severe rash, swelling of the throat, and difficulty breathing may occur. Anaphylactic shock may even take place, during which the blood pressure drops dangerously low and results in dizziness and possibly collapse. If allergic symptoms are significant, contact a doctor immediately.

OTC REMEDIES

There are no OTC products that are recommended for the relief of food allergy symptoms. To alleviate your allergy, it is most important to eliminate the irritating substance from your diet. See the following "Natural Remedies" section for information on this process.

NATURAL REMEDIES

Food allergies can sometimes be identified and alleviated by making dietary changes. If unsure about which foods you may be allergic to, make a list of all the foods and beverages that you consume on a regular basis (foods you eat at least four days per week), the foods you crave, and the foods to which you suspect you may be allergic. Then, an "elimination/rotation/add-back" dietary strategy can be highly effective. Eliminate these foods for two weeks and adhere to a diet of simply-prepared, diversified meals made up of whole, pure foods. Keep notes as to how these dietary changes affect you. After two weeks, reintroduce the foods from your original list—one at a time—into your diet, over the course of four days. Note any allergic reactions that may occur. After identifying the foods that are allergy-promoting, eliminate them completely from your diet for a period of several months. Afterwards, slowly introduce these foods back into the diet by rotating them in small amounts—that is, do not eat them more than once in any four- to seven-day period.

Many people who are allergic to yeast or wheat are not aware that alcoholic beverages containing these ingredients may be contributing to their condition. In fact, most alcoholic beverages do contain yeast or wheat. Thus, in addition to making the dietary changes suggested above, eliminating alcohol may be necessary.

The Five-A-Day Diet (see page 21) can be very helpful in alleviating symptoms of food allergies.

Furthermore, a good multivitamin/mineral will aid in reducing food allergy reactions (see page 14). And the following regimen of natural immune boosters may help to restore and enhance your health. *It is important to note that while certain herbal regimens help maintain a healthy immune system, people with autoimmune illnesses, such as lupus, and those with progressive diseases, such as tuberculosis and multiple sclerosis, should not use herbs for the immune system without consulting their physicians.*

Natural Immune Booster	Dosage	Comments
Astragalus	*During allergy repercussions:* (3) 500-mg capsules/tablets, 3 times daily; *For maintenance:* (3) 500-mg tablets/capsules, daily	A Chinese remedy used for thousands of years; a proven immune stimulant.
Cat's claw	20 to 60 mg, daily	Use standardized extract. Among other functions, it serves as an anti-inflammatory and reduces intestinal problems. Pregnant and lactating women should not take this herb.
Siberian ginseng (*Eleutherococcus senticosus*)	300 to 400 mg, daily	Use standardized extract. Enhances energy and well-being. Do not use this herb if you suffer from any of the following: heart disorder; high blood pressure; hypoglycemia.

Garlic	1 clove, daily, or equivalent dosage in capsules/tablets	Enteric coated tablets standardized to allicin potential are preferable.
Green tea	3 to 4 cups tea daily, or the equivalent in capsules/tablets that provide over 70-percent polyphenols	Available in decaffeinated form. One of the best immune boosters and antiaging foods. Green tea has been shown to reduce the risk of certain types of cancer.
Shiitake	1,000 mg LEM, daily	LEM (lentinan edodes myceli-um) is an extract of the shiitake mushroom that is most potent.

Food Poisoning

Each year, millions of Americans experience moderate to severe food poisoning, as well as hundreds of millions of cases of diarrhea as the result of very mild food poisoning. The actual incidence of this condition is not known because many people mistake it for the flu. *Salmonella* bacteria are the most frequent cause of food poisoning. These bacteria are easily transmitted during the food preparation process, at home or when eating out. The signs of salmonella poisoning can range from simple abdominal cramps to a raging fever. The first symptom is usually diarrhea. Chicken, eggs, beef, and pork products are common sources of salmonella poisoning.

If symptoms are mild, you can self-manage your illness with OTCs and natural remedies. But with any incidence, it is wisest to call a doctor or a pharmacist for advice. The symptoms of food poisoning occur quickly and sometimes very severely. For emergency situations, keep the phone number of the nearest Poison Control Center and hospital emergency room by the telephone. If children are home alone, confirm that they know who to call in case of food poisoning.

For more information, please refer to the individual sections on the specific symptoms you are experiencing, such as fever, headaches, diarrhea, etc. And remember, the best decision is to contact your medical doctor or pharmacist.

Gas

See also Indigestion.

Gas in the digestive tract is usually present as a result of swallowed air. This may occur when someone is eating or drinking too quickly. Also, some people swallow air when they are anxious. Most of the time, swallowed air is released through belching. Some swallowed air passes into the intestines and is released through the anus. Gas may also be produced by particular foods, such as beans, certain fruits and vegetables, and foods with a large amount of indigestible carbohydrates. People with lactose intolerance (see page 238) or who absorb foods poorly are also prone to develop gas. Finally, gum chewing, smoking, and improper swallowing increase gas.

It is generally believed that excessive gas in the intestinal tract causes abdominal pain, bloating, belching, and flatulence. However, it remains uncertain whether the gas itself induces these symptoms or if the people who frequently experience gas may simply have hypersensitive intestines that are inflicted with gas and the other symptoms concurrently. Excessive gas symptoms are influenced by stress and emotional factors, and they overlap with many other conditions (for example, irritable bowel syndrome).

In general, gas problems are resolved naturally, and some OTC products may help bring symptomatic relief. While gas itself is usually not a serious problem, see your doctor if it is accompanied by severe stomach pain or if pain lasts for more than three days.

Repeated belching, called *aerophagia*, is usually caused by unconscious, incorrect breathing of air into the esophagus. When this is the case, a person can belch on command and even produce a series of belches. Education on behavior modification will help; medications are not needed.

OTC REMEDIES

The products listed in the following table provide symptomatic relief from gas problems. Always read the label before using a product.

OTC Remedy	Dosage	Comments
DiGel Antacid/Antigas Tablets/Liquid	As directed on label.	Antacid ingredients neutralize some of the stomach's hydrochloric acid and decrease pepsin (a digestive enzyme) activity. Antigas ingredients act to reduce gas bubbles in the stomach. Can cause a chalky taste in the

		mouth. Some individuals experience mild constipation, stool changes, and heightened thirst. These side effects should not cause significant problems. Do not take if the calcium level in your blood is high.
Gas-X Tablets	As directed on label.	Also available in extra strength. Reduces gas bubbles in the stomach.
Gelusil Sodium Free Liquid/ Tablets	As directed on label.	Also available in extra strength. Same comments as *DiGel* products.
Maalox Anti-Gas Tablets	As directed on label.	Also available in extra strength. Reduces gas bubbles in the stomach.
Mylanta Liquid/Tablets	As directed on label.	Also available in double strength. Neutralize some of the stomach's hydrochloric acid and decrease pepsin (a digestive enzyme) activity. Can cause a chalky taste in mouth. Some individuals experience mild constipation, stool changes, and heightened thirst. These side effects should not cause significant problems. Do not take if the calcium level in your blood is high.

If you have questions or concerns regarding the safety and effectiveness of any product, consult your doctor or pharmacist. Valid concerns have been expressed by authorities in the consumer-health field regarding products that contain certain chemicals. The following warnings have been issued:

- Products containing only aluminum hydroxide or magnesium hydroxide are safe only for limited use.

- Do not use products containing only simethicone, or products containing a combination of magnesium hydroxide, aluminum hydroxide, and simethicone.

NATURAL REMEDIES

Observe your eating habits. Simple alterations in chewing, swallowing, and other eating habits may prevent excessive gas. Also, make mealtime a relaxing, pleasant occasion. Allow enough time to eat properly and to enjoy the food. If you suffer from a lot of gas, consider avoiding sugar because it can be problematic, depending on what is in the stomach at the time. Eliminate carbonated beverages and beer from your diet, as well.

For treating gas and related gastrointestinal problems, several herbs can be of help: chamomile, goldenseal, papaya, and peppermint. These herbs are easily found in local drug stores and health-food markets. You may find the teas of these herbs especially soothing. Chamomile should not be taken continually for long periods of time, and those who are allergic to ragweed should not take chamomile. Furthermore, do not take goldenseal daily for more than a week, and do not take it at all if you are pregnant. People who are allergic to ragweed should use goldenseal with caution.

Parsley is a wonderful natural remedy for the symptoms of indigestion, including gas. Take $1/4$ teaspoon of dried parsley, or several sprigs of the fresh plant. Finally, the products listed in the following table are natural substances that may further help you to prevent gas.

Natural Remedy	Dosage	Comments
Beano	5 drops, added to the food itself before eating, not before cooking	Contains a natural food enzyme that can be very helpful in relieving gas when you know what food is causing the discomfort (for example, broccoli).
BeSure	1 to 2 tablets, with food	Contains a natural food enzyme that can be very helpful in reducing gas in the digestive system. It functions like *Beano* (see above), but comes in tablet form.
Proteolytic enzymes (food enzymes)	Follow directions on label.	Take with a meal. If having only a snack, take half of the recommended dosage. These enzymes help the body to break down protein so that it can be efficiently absorbed. This reduces gas and bloating. You can also take *pancreatin*, a food enzyme that is readily available in drug stores and serves the same functions as the multiple-enzyme products. These supplements are not for children.
Vitamin-B complex*	25 to 50 mg, daily	The B vitamins are necessary for proper digestion of food.

* It is important that the discussed nutrients be part of a basic vitamin/mineral regimen so that the total daily amount of each nutrient obtained from both a multivitamin/mineral and other supplements is approximately the dosage indicated above.

Fungal Infection

See Athlete's Foot; Jock Itch.

Gingivitis

See Dental Problems.

Gum Disease

See Dental Problems.

Hair and Scalp Problems

See also Dandruff; "Seborrhea" under Dermatitis.

There are several conditions that can be considered hair and scalp problems, including baldness, scalp itch, dandruff, and lice. Baldness, or *alopecia*, is influenced by many factors. In both men and women, the following conditions/situations can cause hair loss: poor circulation; skin disease; treatment of illness by surgery, radiation, or chemotherapy; stress; and poor diet. For men, age, heredity, and hormones are usually involved in baldness that is not associated with nutritional or medical conditions. Hair loss in women differs somewhat; even when hair loss in women is similar to "male pattern baldness," it is generally not as severe and most often occurs after menopause. Women may also experience some hair loss after giving birth.

Scalp itch can be the symptom of a number of conditions, including dry skin on the scalp, various rashes, or lice. For information on and remedies for flaking scalp skin, termed dandruff, see the specfic section on that disorder. Head lice are very small parasitic insects that easily spread from individual to individual. The female lays eggs in small sacks that adhere to hairs and hatch within a short period of time. Severe itching results. It is possible to remove these parasites through washing with medicated shampoos. All laundry and personal items must also be cleaned thoroughly.

OTC REMEDIES

The following table lists OTC products available to help combat the hair and scalp problems discussed above. Always read the label before using a product.

OTC Remedy	Application	Comments
For Hair Regrowth		
Rogaine	As directed on label.	May provide some help for a subgroup of men and women with hair loss, notably younger people who have not experienced substantial hair loss. Make sure you are in the subset of people for whom *Rogaine* (minoxidil) is considered effective before purchasing and using the product.
For Scalp Itch		
Cortizone-10 Scalp Itch Liquid	As directed on label.	Do not use if you are allergic to any cortisone products.

For Lice		
A-200 Lice Killing Shampoo	As directed on label.	No common side effects. Do not take if you are allergic to medications that contain any of the following: lindane; pyrethrins; piperonyl butoxide.
Pronto Lice Killing Shampoo & Conditioner	As directed on label.	Same comments as *A-200 Lice Killing Shampoo.*
RID Lice Killing Shampoo	As directed on label.	Same comments as *A-200 Lice Killing Shampoo.*

NATURAL REMEDIES

Stress, poor diet, and vitamin deficiencies are linked to hair loss in some people. Stress-reduction techniques, such as yoga and meditation, and improved nutrition can help reduce or even eliminate some cases of hair loss. Brewer's yeast has been linked with healthier hair growth, as have been sunflower seeds and walnuts. The nutrient biotin may also be helpful. Biotin is essential for healthy skin and hair, and may even help prevent hair loss. Recommended biotin-rich foods include brown rice, bulgur, green peas, lentils, oats, and soybeans. Biotin supplements are another option; see the table below. Also listed are other supplements to consider.

Natural Remedy	Dosage	Comments
Biotin	50 mg, 2 times daily	Deficiencies are linked with skin problems and loss of hair. Take in addition to inositol (see below).

CoQ$_{10}$ (coenzyme Q$_{10}$, also called ubiquinone)	60 mg, daily	Improves circulation to the scalp and increases the amount of oxygen in tissues throughout the body.
Inositol	100 mg, 2 times daily	This substance is essential for hair growth. Take in addition to biotin (see above).
Folic acid	400 mcg, daily	Part of the B-complex family that may be helpful in maintaining healthy hair.
Multivitamin/ mineral*	See pages 14 to 20.	See pages 14 to 20.
Vitamin C*	500 mg, 2 times daily	Improves circulation to the scalp.
Vitamin E*	400 IU, daily	Take with a meal. Mixed tocopherols supplying 400 IU of d-alpha tocopherol are preferred. Can be used for long-term maintenance. Improves circulation to the scalp; enhances health of the hair and its growth.
Zinc*	30 mg, daily	Take with a meal. Stimulates hair growth. Doses in excess of 100 mg can depress immune function. Zinc lozenges are an option for easy intake and good absorption.

* It is important that the discussed nutrients be part of a basic vitamin/mineral regimen so that the total daily amount of each nutrient obtained from both a multivitamin/mineral and other supplements is approximately the dosage indicated above.

Halitosis

See Bad Breath.

Headache

See also Migraine.

About 75 percent of Americans have at least one headache per year. Furthermore, approximately 45 million Americans have chronic headaches. The pain associated with a headache can range from dull and throbbing to sharp and stabbing. There may be pain on only one or on both sides of the head. The average headache lasts for five hours.

Tension is the cause of the vast majority of headaches. Repressed emotions (for example, anger and fear) may also play a role in the onset of headaches. Sometimes they may be related to other health problems, such as arthritis, constipation, hypertension, head injury, or eye, ear, and throat disorders. In addition, certain foods or food additives may cause headaches in some individuals—for example, alcohol; caffeine; chocolate; dairy products; fermented foods; marinated foods; vinegar; MSG; and sulfites. Other triggers for headaches include: stress on the job or at home; fatigue; pollution; allergies; vitamin deficiencies; and grinding of the teeth (*See* Bruxism, page 107).

While most headaches can be safely and effectively treated with OTCs and natural remedies, consult a physician if headaches are disrupting your regular activities or if you experience any of the following: blurred vision; light sensitivity; visual color changes; pressure in the facial/sinus area; a pounding heart; throbbing in the head and temples that makes you feel like your head might explode. Pay special attention if headaches recur after the age of forty, if they get stronger or occur more frequently, if they change location, or if they are accompanied by numbness, dizziness, or memory loss.

OTC REMEDIES

The products listed in the following chart are analgesics—substances that relieve or reduce pain. If you have experienced side effects from any nonprescription pain relievers, do not take any of these remedies without consulting your doctor. Always read the label before using a product.

OTC Remedy	Dosage	Comments
Acetaminophen *Excedrin Aspirin-Free; Panadol; Tylenol*	325 mg regular strength; generally, 500 mg extra strength	Do not drink alcohol and use products containing acetaminophen. The combination can cause liver damage. Do not take with other analgesics. Some of these products, such as *Tylenol,* are available in regular, junior, and extra strength.
Aspirin (acetylsalicylic acid) *Ascriptin; Bayer; Bufferin; Ecotrin; Empirin; Excedrin Extra Strength*	325 mg regular strength; generally, 500 mg extra strength	If pregnant, consult your doctor before taking products containing aspirin. Do not take products containing aspirin during the last three months of pregnancy. Children and teens should not use products containing aspirin

		for colds, flus, or chickenpox. Do not take products containing aspirin if you have asthma, stomach problems, gastric ulcers, bleeding problems, or if you are allergic to aspirin.
Ibuprofen *Advil; Arthritis Foundation Ibuprofen; Motrin IB; Nuprin*	200 mg	If pregnant, consult your doctor before taking this remedy. Do not take products containing this ingredient during the last three months of pregnancy. Do not take this ingredient if you are allergic to aspirin. Do not take this ingredient with any other analgesics. Consult your doctor before taking this remedy with prescription drugs.
Ketoprofen *Orudis KT*	12.5 mg	Same comments as Ibuprofen.
Naproxen sodium *Aleve*	220 mg	If pregnant, consult your doctor before taking this remedy. Do not take products containing this ingredient during the last three months of pregnancy. Do not take this ingredient with any other analgesics. Consult your doctor before taking this remedy with prescription drugs.

When used responsibly, acetaminophen, aspirin, ibuprofen, ketoprofen, and naproxen sodium are safe and effective. Look for single-ingredient products. Some headache remedies contain ingredients, such as caffeine, that may aggravate your condition. If you have questions or concerns regarding the safety and effectiveness of any product, consult your doctor or pharmacist. Also, keep in mind that OTCs are very helpful for some types of headaches, but natural approaches may be the answer for preventing migraine-type headaches.

NATURAL REMEDIES

Diet may play a role in your headaches. Establish a healthy, balanced diet for yourself, such as the Five-A-Day Diet (see page 21). Also, take a multivitamin/ mineral that provides the supplementation outlined in the table below. Furthermore, be sure to get adequate rest; fatigue can leave your head very achy.

Find out if you have any food allergies, which can bring on severe headaches. Follow the dietary advice discussed in the "Natural Remedies" section under *Food Allergy* to determine if you may be allergic to any foods that you consume on a regular basis. The most common foods to bring on a migraine attack are chocolate, cheese, and alcohol. There is some evidence that lowering dietary-fat intake can decrease the incidence of migraines. See the section on migraine (page 247) for more information.

Sometimes headaches are stress-related. Many people have found that the following alternative approaches bring relief: biofeedback; massage; and meditation and relaxation techniques, including deep-breathing and yoga. For the treatment of migraine headaches, chiropractic and acupuncture are also frequently effective.

Most simply, resting in a dark, quiet room and

applying ice to the painful area can relieve a headache. Also, certain natural substances and supplements have proven beneficial in the treatment of headaches. See the following table for more information.

Natural Remedy	Dosage	Comments
Feverfew *Mygrafew*	125 mg, 2 times daily	To prevent migraine headaches, take this substance on a daily basis. Make sure the product contains at least 0.2-percent parthenolide. Also note the expiration date on the bottle. Parthenolide is relatively unstable; the closer the product gets to the expiration date, the less likely it is there will be enough parthenolide present for the product to be effective.
Ginkgo biloba	Up to 240 mg, daily	Use a standardized extract containing 24 percent ginkgo-flavone glycosides and 6-percent terpene lactones. May be beneficial in preventing migraine due to its ability to inhibit platelet activating factor. Ginkgo can cause minor headaches when initially taken. This effect subsides usually within the first week of use.
Kava kava	140 to 210 mg of kava-lactones	Kava has a mellowing effect and may be helpful for the treatment of stress-related headaches.
Multivitamin/ mineral	See pages 14 to 20.	See pages 14 to 20. Be sure this supplement supplies 400 mg of magnesium and a minimum of 400 mg of calcium.

		Consider that 1,000 mg or more daily of calcium may decrease the incidence of migraine.
Valerian	300 to 500 mg	Use a standardized extract. Traditionally used for relaxation · at bedtime, but may be helpful in reducing the incidence of recurring headaches due to stress. Do not drive a vehicle while under the effects of this herb.

Heartburn

See Indigestion.

Hemorrhoids

See also Varicose Veins.

This condition is characterized by swollen veins around the anus and in the rectal wall. Hemorrhoids are universal; they occur in adults and children, men and women. When they occur without symptoms, they may even be considered normal. Common symptoms of this condition are inflammation, pain, itching, and bleeding, especially after defecation. Hemorrhoids can be caused by many factors, including: prolonged periods of sitting; constipation; poor nutrition; excess weight; heavy lifting; lack of regular physical exercise; birthing a baby; and liver damage. A severe case of hemorrhoids may require surgery, but mild to moderate cases can be managed at home.

OTC REMEDIES

The following table lists several products that provide symptomatic relief from hemorroids. Always read the label before using a product. If there is no improvement after seven days of treatment, see a doctor.

OTC Remedy	Application	Comments
For External Anal Itching		
Anusol HC-1 Anti-Itch Hydrocortisone Ointment	As directed on label.	Reduces inflammation, pain, and itching. Do not use if you have had a negative reaction to any topical anesthetics. No common side effects. Allergic reactions, such as rashes, nervousness, depressed heart rate, dizziness, and vision problems are possible, but unusual. Contact your doctor if you feel adverse effects.
Cortaid Maximum Strength Cream/ Ointment/Spray	As directed on label.	Reduces inflammation. No common side effects. Further irritation of the skin occurs only infrequently. Do not use if you are allergic to any cortisone products.
Cortizone-5 Creme/Ointment	As directed on label.	Same comments as *Cortaid Maximum Strength Cream/ Ointment/Spray.*
Cortizone for Kids Anti-Itch Creme	As directed on label.	Same comments as *Cortaid Maximum Strength Cream/ Ointment/Spray.*
Cortizone-10 Creme/Ointment	As directed on label.	Available in regular and *External Anal-Itch Relief* formulas. Same comments as *Cortaid Maximum Strength Cream/Ointment/Spray.*

Preparation-H Hydrocortisone Anti-Itch Cream	As directed on label.	Reduces inflammation and temporarily anesthetizes the affected area. Do not use if you have had a negative reaction to any topical anesthetic. No common side effects. Allergic reactions, such as ashes, nervousness, depressed heart rate, dizziness, and vision problems are possible, but unusual. Contact your doctor if you feel adverse effects.

For Pain, Soreness, & Burning

Anusol Hemorrhoidal Suppositories	As directed on label.	Reduces inflammation and pain. Discontinue if swelling, redness, pain, or allergic reactions occur. If there is bleeding, see a doctor.
Anusol Ointment	As directed on label.	Reduces inflammation. No common side effects. Further irritation of the skin occurs only infrequently. Do not use if you are allergic to any cortisone products.
Preparation-H Cream/Ointment	As directed on label.	Same comments as *Preparation-H Hydrocortisone Anti-Itch Cream.*
Preparation-H Suppositories	As directed on label.	Same comments as *Anusol Hemorrhoidal Suppositories.*
Tronolane Anesthetic Cream for Hemorrhoids	As directed on label.	Same comments as *Preparation-H Hydrocortisone Anti-Itch Cream.*
Tronolane Hemorrhoidal Suppositories	As directed on label.	Same comments as *Anusol Hemorrhoidal Suppositories.*
Tucks Clear Hemorrhoidal Gel	As directed on label.	Same comments as *Preparation-H Hydrocortisone Anti-Itch Cream.*

Tucks Pre-Moistened Hemorrhoidal/ Vaginal Pads	As directed on label.	Same comments as *Anusol Hemorrhoidal Suppositories.*

NATURAL REMEDIES

Hemorrhoids can be both avoided and treated by following a regular exercise program, by drinking six to eight glasses of water daily, and by eating a diet that is rich in whole grains and high-fiber foods. You may want to try the Five-A-Day Diet (see page 21) or another diet recommended by a trained nutritionist. Healthy eating, exercise, and stress management will avoid constipation and, therefore, straining when moving the bowels. Finally, the table below lists several natural substances that will help to prevent hemorrhoids.

Natural Remedy	Dosage	Comments
Vitamin C*	500 mg, 2 times daily	Helps to maintain a healthy vascular system.
Horse chestnut extract *Venostat*	35 to 70 mg, daily	Standardized to aescin content. This extract is rich in specific bioflavonoids and shown to increase the tone of veins, which prevents them from expanding to form hemorrhoids.
Grape-seed extract or **Pine bark extract** *Pycnogenol*	50 mg, daily	Use standardized extract. Helps to strengthen the veins and capillaries. Grape-seed extract and pine bark extract are comparable substances.
Multivitamin/ mineral*	See pages 14 to 20.	See pages 14 to 20.

Vitamin A*	10,000 IU, daily	An important vitamin for the development and health of vein, artery, and capillary linings. Take with a meal. Can be toxic when taken in large amounts for a long period of time.

* It is important that the discussed nutrients be part of a basic vitamin/mineral regimen so that the total daily amount of each nutrient obtained from both a multivitamin/mineral and other supplements is approximately the dosage indicated above.

Herpesvirus

The herpes simplex virus (HSV) causes infections that are characterized by single cold sores or multiple clusters of cold sores, skin eruptions, or lesions. These areas are filled with a clear fluid, inflamed, and slightly raised from the skin surface. After infection, the virus never leaves. It can remain dormant for years. Stress and illness are associated with outbreaks. For reasons unknown, the virus almost never recurs after the age of fifty.

The sores associated with herpes commonly appear around the mouth, the lips, the conjunctiva and cornea of the eye, and the genitals. There are two types of this virus: HSV-1 (oral herpes) and HSV-2. Cold sores and skin eruptions indicate HSV-1. This virus can infect the cornea of the eye. Infection of the eye is extremely serious and requires immediate attention by a physician. HSV-1 can also cause encephalitis, an infection of the brain.

HSV-2, or genital herpes, is the most widespread form of herpes. It is transmitted sexually. HSV-2 can be transmitted to infants at birth, possibly causing blindness, brain damage, and even death. Some people who have HSV-2 remain symptomless, while others suffer frequent outbreaks and even more serious conditions, such as liver inflammation. Symptoms include sores within a week of exposure; painful blisters around the genitals and/or the mouth that are infectious for up to twenty-one days; blisters on the groin, scrotum, and penis; or a burning or tingling in the vaginal area, followed by blisters in the rectal, vaginal, clitoral, and cervical areas. There may be pain on urination and a watery discharge from the urethra in both men and women. The blisters eventually yield pus, crust over, and heal, leaving no scarring.

This condition requires a doctor's attention. Do not self-diagnose herpes. Once you have received a doctor's guidance on how to manage the virus, discuss the products listed under "OTC Remedies" and the supplements suggested under "Natural Remedies." They may be helpful in reducing growth of the herpesvirus. It is important to avoid activities that can spread this virus until the condition is clearly resolved.

OTC REMEDIES

The OTC products listed in the following chart are formulated to prevent the outbreak of or relieve the symptoms of herpes. Always read the label before using a product.

OTC Remedy	Dosage	Comments
Herp-Eeze	2 capsules, daily,	Take on an empty stomach. An herbal extract that may be helpful in preventing herpes outbreak.
Herpecin L	Apply to lips every hour during outdoor exposure.	Helps treat and prevent lip-cracking due to sun exposure. May not necessarily inhibit herpesvirus.

NATURAL REMEDIES

Consult your physician before trying any approach. After talking with your doctor, consider avoiding foods that are high in arginine, such as peanuts, most nuts, chocolate, barley, corn, and oats. Arginine nourishes the virus. To ease pain and suffering in the genital area, use ice packs. Also, for itching and pain, try warm Epsom salt baths. In addition, the following table lists several natural substances that may strengthen your defense against the virus.

Natural Remedy	Dosage	Comments
Bioflavonoids	60 mg, daily	May help prevent herpesvirus growth.
Grape-seed extract	25 to 50 mg, daily	May help prevent herpesvirus growth.
Lysine	*At the first sign of an outbreak:* 1,000 mg, 3 times daily, for five days; *For maintenance:* 500 to 1,000 mg, daily	A natural amino acid that competes with arginine and helps to deny it access to the virus.
Multivitamin/ mineral*	See pages 14 to 20.	See pages 14 to 20.

Vitamin C*	1,000 mg, 3 times daily	Helps maintain the immune system. Safe for long-term maintenance.
Vitamin E*	400 IU, daily	Take with a meal. Promotes healing and may prevent the spread of infection.
Zinc*	Up to 50 mg, daily	Take with a meal. Helps maintain the immune system. Doses in excess of 100 mg can depress immune function.

* It is important that the discussed nutrients be part of a basic vitamin/mineral regimen so that the total daily amount of each nutrient obtained from both a multivitamin/mineral and other supplements is approximately the dosage indicated above.

High Cholesterol

Cholesterol is a fat-like substance found throughout the body and in food products that come from animals. It is part of the lipid family. Cholesterol plays a role in the structure of the brain and nerve cells. Actually, it is present and necessary in every cell. But excess cholesterol in the blood has been associated with an increased risk of heart disease. The plaques that narrow the arteries and often lead to heart attacks and strokes are largely composed of cholesterol. Therefore, measures should be taken to keep blood cholesterol down to a healthy level.

The cholesterol ingested through foods does influence the level of cholesterol in the blood somewhat, so a high-cholesterol diet should be avoided. But this influence is rather minimal in most people. It is a minority of people (about one-third of the population) whose blood cholesterol reaches dangerously high levels from dietary cholesterol. The intake of fats, especially saturated fat, plays a far greater role in elevating blood-cholesterol levels, as the body makes cholesterol from fats. A sedentary lifestyle and excess weight are also dangerous contributors to the production of high cholesterol in the blood.

OTC REMEDIES

Metamucil is an OTC product that contains natural fiber. It is used for restoring and maintaining regularity, but can also be of value in maintaining healthy blood-cholesterol levels.

NATURAL REMEDIES

One of the most important ways to maintain a healthy blood-cholesterol level is to follow a low-fat (especially a low-saturated-fat), low-cholesterol diet. Meat and dairy products are the primary sources of dietary cholesterol. Vegetables, fruits, and grains have absolutely no cholesterol. Furthermore, they can help lower cholesterol due to fiber content, as well as prevent the cholesterol produced in the body from being converted (oxidized) into a damaging form. Cold-water fish, dried beans, garlic, and olive oil are helpful in keeping the body's cholesterol at a healthy level.

In addition to diet, a good exercise and stress-reduction program can reduce cholesterol levels and, therefore, the risk of heart disease in general. It appears that adequate intake of the antioxidant vitamins C and

E, along with other antioxidants such as grape-seed extract, lutein, and rosemary extract, can prevent the cholesterol produced in the body from being converted to harmful artery-damaging plaque. The table below offers further information.

Natural Remedy	Dosage	Comments
Garlic *Centrum; Garlimax; Garlique; Highgar; Kyolic; Kwai; One A-Day*	1 fresh clove, or the equivalent in capsules/tablets, daily	Serves to lower both cholesterol and high blood pressure. The most researched products include the enteric-coated *Kwai* tablets, which release garlic into the small intestine to maximize absorption of the active constituents, and the well-tested *Kyolic* tablets. Note, onion may be equally beneficial, but does not have the clinical results to support claims at this time.
Multivitamin/ mineral with antioxidants	See pages 14 to 20.	See pages 14 to 20.
Red Yeast *Cholestin*	2 capsules, 2 times daily.	A natural yeast, grown on rice, that contains a small amount of lovastatin and other compounds shown to lower cholesterol. If you have any pre-existing liver condition or if you are taking prescription medications, do not use without consulting a physician.
Tocotrienols *Evolve*	1 to 2 capsules, daily	A rice bran derivative related to vitamin E. May be helpful in lowering/maintaining healthy cholesterol levels.

Indigestion

See also Gas.

Indigestion, also called *dyspepsia*, can be a condition in itself or it can be a symptom of another illness. Symptoms of indigestion include: heartburn; gas and belching; nausea and vomiting; a bloated feeling; and stomach pain. It might be caused by gastritis—an inflammation of the stomach or intestinal lining—or by a gastric (stomach) ulcer. Usually, however, indigestion is due to some simple interference with normal stomach functioning, caused by one or more of the following: overeating; poor diet; drinking fluids while eating; swallowing air and/or talking while eating; chewing with an open mouth; gulping food and rushing meals; drugs; heavy smoking; alcohol; and/or emotional upset from anger, fear, or worry. Food allergies can be culprits, as well as stress. And for some people, carbohydrates, in particular, cause indigestion and gas.

Acid indigestion is a common discomfort that can involve: gaseousness; a feeling of fullness; gnawing or burning pain localized in the upper abdomen; nausea; vomiting; belching; burning sensations in the gastrointestinal tract; and, after eating, a change in bowel habits. Heartburn is a more specific condition, defined as an irritation of the esophagus by stomach acid. The stomach uses hydrochloric acid in digestion. Sometimes this acid "backs up" into the esophagus and produces that characteristic burning. Certain foods and substances can cause heartburn, such as: chocolate; citrus fruits; fatty, spicy, fried, and tomato-based foods; alcohol; and coffee. It can also be the result of stress, or it can be a telltale sign of other disorders, such as ulcers, hiatal hernias, and allergies.

Peptic and esophageal ulcers, which are sores in the linings of the stomach and esophagus respectively, happen when the tissue is eaten away by stomach acid and digestive juices. A hiatal hernia occurs when a small section of the stomach bulges up over the diaphragm, instead of remaining in normal position in the abdomen. You should see a doctor if you suspect any of these conditions. Also, sometimes what is called heartburn may actually be a symptom of heart disease or a gallbladder problem. So if heartburn is a persistent symptom, it is very important to consult a physican.

OTC REMEDIES

The OTC products listed in the following chart are formulated to relieve the symptoms of indigestion. Always read the label before using a product.

OTC Remedy	Dosage	Comments
For Relief From Acid Indigestion and Heartburn		
Alka-Seltzer Antacid & Pain Reliever (contains aspirin)	As directed on label.	Antacid ingredients neutralize some of the stomach's hydrochloric acid and decrease pepsin (a digestive enzyme) activity. If pregnant, consult your doctor before taking products containing aspirin during the last three months of pregnancy.

		Children and teens should not use products containing aspirin for colds, flus, or chickenpox. Do not take products containing aspirin if you have asthma, stomach problems, gastric ulcers, bleeding problems, or if you are allergic to aspirin.
DiGel Antacid/Antigas Tablets/Liquid	As directed on label.	Antacid ingredients neutralize some of the stomach's hydrochloric acid and decrease pepsin (a digestive enzyme) activity. Antigas ingredients act to reduce gas bubbles in the stomach. Can cause a chalky taste in mouth. Some individuals experience mild constipation, stool changes, and heightened thirst. These side effects should not cause significant problems. Do not take if the calcium level in your blood is high or if you are allergic to any antacids.
Gaviscon Antacid Tablets	As directed on label.	Also available in extra strength. Neutralize some of the stomach's hydrochloric acid and decreases pepsin (a digestive enzyme) activity. Can cause a chalky taste in mouth. Some individuals experience mild constipation, stool changes, and heightened thirst. These side effects should not cause significant problems. Do not take if the calcium level in your blood is high or if you are allergic to any antacids.
Gelusil Sodium Free Tablets/Liquid	As directed on label.	Also available in extra strength. Same comments as *DiGel* products.
Pepcid AC	As directed on label.	Prevents the release of

		histamine, thus reducing the stomach's secretion of acid. No common side effects. Some individuals experience dizziness, headache, and diarrhea, but these effects are unusual.
Phillips' Milk of Magnesia Antacids	As directed on label.	Neutralizes some of the stomach's hydrochloric acid and decreases pepsin (a digestive enzyme) activity. Can cause a chalky taste in mouth. Some individuals experience mild constipation, stool changes, and heightened thirst. These side effects should not cause significant problems. Do not take if the calcium level in your blood is high or if you are allergic to any antacids.
Rolaids Antacid Tablets	As directed on label.	Also available in *Calcium Rich/ Sodium Free* form. Same comments as *Phillips' Milk of Magnesia Antacids*. Concerning the *Calcium Rich* formula, do not take if you are allergic to calcium or if the level of calcium in your blood is high. There are no common side effects associated with calcium supplements. Possible side effects that occur only infrequently include: digestive problems; headaches; dry mouth; feelings of weakness; and appetitite reduction.
Tagamet HB	As directed on label.	Same comments as *Pepcid AC*.
Zantac 75	As directed on label.	Same comments as *Pepcid AC*.
For Relief From Acid Indigestion		
Mylanta Tablets/ Liquid	As directed on label.	Also available in double strength. Neutralizes some of the stomach's hydrochloric acid

		and decreases pepsin (a digestive enzyme) activity. Can cause a chalky taste in mouth. Some individuals experience mild constipation, stool changes, and heightened thirst. These side effects should not cause significant problems. Do not take if the calcium level in your blood is high.
Tums *Antacid Tablets*	As directed on label.	Available in various strengths, including regular, *Tums E-X*, and *Tums Ultra*. Same comments as *Phillips' Milk of Magnesia Antacids*. *Tums* products provide calcium. Do not take if you are allergic to calcium or if the level of calcium in your blood is high. There are no common side effects associated with calcium supplements. Possible side effects that occur only infrequently include: digestive problems; headaches; dry mouth; feelings of weakness; and appetitite reduction.

For Relief From Heartburn

Maalox *Heartburn* *Relief Tablets*	As directed on label.	Neutralize some of the stomach's hydrochloric acid and decrease pepsin (a digestive enzyme) activity. Can cause a chalky taste in mouth. Some individuals experience mild constipation, stool changes, and heightened thirst. These side effects should not cause significant problems. Do not take if the calcium level in your blood is high or if you are allergic to any antacids.

Pepto-Bismol Original Tablets/ Caplets/Liquid	As directed on label.	Common side effects include dark stools and tongue. These effects are harmless. The same warnings given for use of aspirin apply here: If pregnant, consult your doctor before taking products. Do not take products during the last three months of pregnancy. Children and teens should not use for colds, flus, or chickenpox. Do not give to a child with a fever. Do not take products if you have asthma, stomach problems, gastric ulcers, bleeding problems, or if you are allergic to aspirin.

It is important to note that over-the-counter drugs may relieve symptoms of acid indigestion or heartburn but can sometimes interfere with digestion. If you have questions or concerns regarding the safety and effectiveness of any product, consult your doctor or pharmacist. Also, valid concerns have been expressed by authorities in the consumer-health field regarding the safety and effectiveness of products containing certain chemicals. The following warning has been issued:

• Products containing only aluminum hydroxide or magnesium hydroxide should be taken for limited use only.

NATURAL REMEDIES

Before trying OTC products to relieve indigestion, you may want to drink some chamomile tea to settle the stomach. This natural remedy may be just what you need. Drinking a large glass of water at the first sign of heartburn, avoiding stress, and not lying down immediately after eating are other healthy and helpful practices. Proper eating habits, investigation of possible food allergies (see page 188), and stress management may alleviate digestive problems, as well. Learn to relax while you eat, and manage your time more efficiently. It is important to chew food well and to eat slowly. Also, try taking a nice walk around the block to aid digestion after a meal, rather than retiring to a comfy chair or couch.

If heartburn occurs primarily in the evening, make your last meal of the day high in carbohydrates and low in protein, especially animal protein. High protein intake causes an increase in acid production and can heighten the risk of heartburn. An added benefit of following this advice is that a dinner high in carbohydrates facilitates better sleep. Also, try juicing a potato (the entire potato, including the skin), mixing the juice with the same amount of water, and drinking it immediately, three times per day. This remedy has been known to bring relief.

Simple dietary modifications may resolve indigestion without the use of OTCs. Eat well-balanced meals that are rich in fiber. Reduce your salt intake, and avoid the following: white sugar; bakery products; pasta; processed, spicy, highly-seasoned, fried, junk, and fatty foods; red meat; carbonated beverages; caffeine; alcohol; chocolate and other candies; peanuts; dairy products; citrus juices; tomatoes; seasoning pepper; and beans. Find out which foods cause you particular trouble with digestion, then avoid these foods or combinations that contain them. For example, some people get indigestion from mixing sweet foods, such as fruit, sugary rolls, desserts, etc., with protein. Furthermore, consume plenty of whole, unprocesssed foods, being sure to include lots of fruits and vegetables in your diet. Especially helpful fruits are papayas, kiwis, and pineapples, because they contain enzymes—for example, papain from papaya, and bromelain from pineapple—that aid digestion. These enzymes are available in supplement form as well. Pancreatin supplements, which are preparations of pancreatic enzymes, may be even more effective, since enzymes from the pancreas play a role in the digestion of fats, starch, and protein. See the following table for more information.

Physicians sometimes prescribe natural hydrochloric acid supplements for acid indigestion. This may sound like it would add fuel to the fire, but the truth is that your doctor may determine that your indigestion is actually due to low stomach acid, a common occurrence in the senior population.

Natural Remedy	Dosage	Comments
Acidophilus capsules/tablets (*Lactobacillus acidophilus*)	2 to 4 capsules/ tablets, 3 times daily	Helps restore friendly bacteria in the gut. Only purchase products that have been refrigerated, to ensure and maintain activity.
Bromelain	500 MCU, 4 times daily	An enzyme that aids digestion, particularly helping the body to break down and absorb protein. If MCU activity is not stated on the label, the product may lack potency.

Hydrochloric acid *Acidulin*	300 to 600 mg (usually 1 to 2 capsules/tablets)	Take before meal. Try with one meal, and if it aggravates the condition, discontinue using and consult your physician. Supplements may be labeled *glutamic acid HCL*.
Pancreatin	250 to 500 mg	Take before meal. An enzyme that can help break down proteins.

Inflammation

Any part of the body—internal areas or external areas—can experience inflammation. This condition is characterized by swelling, pain, and a rise in body temperature in the affected area. Bacterial infection is a common cause of inflammation, especially internal inflammation. However, the condition can also be initiated by trauma, strain, or an illness, such as arthritis. (Bacterial arthritis with inflammation is often coupled with an infection of the gallbladder, kidneys, or lungs.)

Heat and cold therapies may help, as may rest and medication. If the condition persists, see a doctor.

OTC REMEDIES

The products listed in the following chart are analgesics—substances that work to relieve or reduce pain. These products also combat fever. If you have experienced side effects from any nonprescription pain relievers, do not take any of these remedies without consulting your doctor. Always read the label before using a product.

OTC Remedy	Dosage	Comments
Acetaminophen *Excedrin Aspirin-Free; Panadol; Tylenol*	325 mg regular strength; generally, 500 mg extra strength	Do not drink alcohol and use products containing acetaminophen. The combination can cause liver damage. Do not take with other analgesics. Some of these products, such as *Tylenol,* are available in regular, junior, and extra strength.
Aspirin (acetylsalicylic acid) *Ascriptin; Bayer; Bufferin; Ecotrin; Empirin; Excedrin Extra Strength*	325 mg regular strength; generally, 500 mg extra strength	If pregnant, consult your doctor before taking products containing aspirin. Do not take products containing aspirin during the last three months of pregnancy. Children and teens should not use products containing aspirin for colds, flus, or chickenpox. Do not take products containing aspirin if you have asthma, stomach problems, gastric ulcers, bleeding problems, or if you are allergic to aspirin.
Ibuprofen *Advil; Arthritis Foundation Ibuprofen; Motrin IB; Nuprin*	200 mg	If pregnant, consult your doctor before taking this remedy. Do not take products containing this ingredient during the last three months of pregnancy. Do not take this ingredient if you are allergic to aspirin. Do not take this ingredient with any other analgesics. Consult your doctor before taking this remedy with prescription drugs.
Ketoprofen *Orudis KT*	12.5 mg	Same comments as Ibuprofen.

Naproxen sodium *Aleve*	220 mg	If pregnant, consult your doctor before taking this remedy. Do not take products containing this ingredient during the last three months of pregnancy. Do not take this ingredient with any other analgesics. Consult your doctor before taking this remedy with prescription drugs.

When used responsibly, acetaminophen, aspirin, ibuprofen, ketoprofen, and naproxen sodium are safe and effective. Look for single-ingredient products. If you have questions or concerns regarding the safety and effectiveness of any product, consult your doctor or pharmacist.

NATURAL REMEDIES

The best way to alleviate the aches and pains associated with long-term inflammation is to follow a diet that is rich in whole foods and that contains five to ten servings of fruits and vegetables per day. The diet should be 75-percent raw foods. Also, avoid colas, sugar, white-flour products, and junk foods. In addition, there are a number of natural substances that reduce the inflammation of joints, especially if the problem is related to wear and tear on the structural components found in the joints. These are listed in the table below.

Natural Remedy	Dosage	Comments
Glucosamine and chondroitin *Osteo Biflex*	Divide up total dosage equal to 1,500 mg of glucosamine, daily. For example, take (3) 250-mg tablets in the morning and (3) 250-mg tablets in the evening.	Be sure to take with meals, to avoid upset stomach. These products are not pain relievers per se, but they stimulate the healthy growth of joint components. Therefore, they should be taken for two months at a minimum.
Hydrolyzed gelatin *Knox Nutra Joint; Arthred G*	Mix 1 scoop in favorite beverage, daily	Natural hydrolyzed collagen (gelatin) material helps to build and maintain healthy joint components. Requires daily use for two months to achieve optimal effect.
Multivitamin/ mineral* including antioxidants	See pages 14 to 20.	See pages 14 to 20.
Vitamin C*	500 mg, 3 times daily	Necessary for collagen synthesis. Safe for long-term maintenance.
Vitamin E*	400 IU, daily	Take with a meal. Inhibits the breakdown of and stimulates the synthesis of cartilage. Mixed tocopherols supplying 400 IU of d-alpha tocopherol are preferred. Can be used for long-term maintenance.

* It is important that the discussed nutrients be part of a basic vitamin/mineral regimen so that the total daily amount of each nutrient obtained from both a multivitamin/mineral and other supplements is approximately the dosage indicated above.

Insect Bites

See also Bee Stings.

Many insects bite or sting, including ants, bees, gnats, mosquitoes, spiders, and wasps, to name a few. Often, insect bites sting, itch, redden, and/or swell. Although an insect bite is usually nothing more than an annoyance, it can sometimes be cause for serious concern. For example, in the United States, a mosquito bite is generally harmless, but in other parts of the world, mosquitoes may carry malaria. And spider bites are most often harmless, but there are several species of poisonous spiders that live in certain regions. So be sure to find out if there are any special precautions that should be taken in your area.

Lyme disease, widely reported in the eastern United States, and Rocky Mountain fever, almost entirely occurring in the western United States, are serious infections caused by tick bites. If left untreated, these diseases can lead to life-long illnesses such as arthritis and even heart disease. If bitten by a tick, it is important to remove the insect gently but swiftly. Speedy removal of the tick can help prevent Lyme disease. It is vital that no part of the tick remains embedded in the skin. If possible, use tweezers and do not touch the tick with your hand. Thoroughly wash the area that has been bitten with soap and water. Do not apply other substances, such as petroleum jelly. If you even suspect that you have been bitten by a tick, consult a physician to make sure you have not contracted Lyme disease, which can be diagnosed and treated to prevent serious complications. A bite by a deer tick, which carries Lyme disease, often is indicated by a white spot at the point of penetration, surrounded by a more extensive circle of redness.

OTC REMEDIES

The following table lists a number of OTC products that are helpful in relieving the itchiness, pain, and swelling associated with insect bites. Always read the label before using a product.

OTC Remedy	Application	Comments
Americaine Topical Anesthetic Spray/First Aid Ointment	As directed on label	Temporarily blocks the pain messages sent from the skin to the brain. Further skin irritation (possibly including hives) due to use of this product is uncommon.
Benadryl Itch-Relief Cream/Spray/Gel	As directed on label.	Also available in maximum-strength and children's formulas. Reduces inflammation. Further skin irritation due to use of this product is uncommon.
BiCozene Creme	As directed on label.	Topical anti-infective. Further skin irritation due to use of this product is uncommon.
Caladryl Lotion	As directed on label.	Also available in a cream for children.

Caldecort *Anti-Itch* *Cream/Spray*	As directed on label.	Also available in *Cream for Kids* formula. Reduces inflammation. Further skin irritation due to use of this product is uncommon. Do not use if you are allergic to any cortisone products.
Cortaid *Cream/Ointment/* *Spray*	As directed on label.	The regular- and maximum-strength formulas are available in cream and ointment forms, while the maximum-strength formula is also available in spray form. Reduces inflammation. Further skin irritation due to use of this product is uncommon. Do not use if you are allergic to any cortisone products.
Cortizone *for Kids* *Anti-Itch Creme*	As directed on label.	Reduces inflammation. Further skin irritation due to use of this product is uncommon. Do not use if you are allergic to any cortisone products.
Cortizone-5 *Creme/Ointment*	As directed on label.	Same comments as *Cortizone for Kids Anti-Itch Creme.*
Cortizone-10 *Creme/Ointment*	As directed on label.	Same comments as *Cortizone for Kids Anti-Itch Creme.*

If you have questions or concerns regarding the safety and effectiveness of any product, consult your doctor or pharmacist.

NATURAL REMEDIES

For common, less serious insect bites, wash the bitten area with soap and water and apply ice to swollen tissue. Afterward, if needed, apply a paste made of baking soda and water to the affected area. Also, meat tenderizer is a helpful substance. With $1/4$ teaspoon of tenderizer and 1 to 2 teaspoons of water, make a paste and apply a small amount. Tenderizer contains papain, an enzyme that helps fight pain.

Insomnia

This condition is characterized by a prolonged period of sleepless nights. Many factors commonly contribute to insomnia: stress; alcohol; caffeine; lack of regular physical exercise; some medications; and illness, such as lung, liver, heart, kidney, and digestive diseases. Some people suffer insomnia due to *sleep apnea*—a disorder that causes a momentary cessation of breathing several times during the night. (Obesity is linked to sleep apnea.) *Ironically, medications used to help a person sleep can often become a cause of insomnia themselves.* If changes in behavior and diet do not resolve insomnia, it is wise to consult a doctor to rule out any underlying illness.

OTC REMEDIES

The following table lists OTC sleep-aid products. Always read the label before using a product.

OTC Remedy	Dosage	Comments
Diphenhydramine hydrochloride *Nytol Quickcaps Caplets; Unisom Maximum Strength Sleepgels*	As directed on label.	Common side effects include dizziness and dryness of the nose, mouth, and throat. More severe side effects, such as vision changes, rashes, and difficulty urinating, occur only infrequently but require a doctor's attention.
Diphenhydramine citrate and magnesium salicylate *Excedrin PM Tablets*	325 mg	Same comments as Diphenhydramine hydrochloride. The following warnings apply to magnesium salicylate: Do not take at the same time as tetracycline medications; allow at least an hour between these medications. Do not take if breastfeeding; avoid taking during pregnancy, or contact a physician beforehand; risk varies with product. Do not take if you have ulcers or bleeding problems; consult with a doctor if you have had ulcers or gout in the past, and if you have asthma or polyps in the nasal passages. Common side effects include indigestion, ringing in the ears, nausea, vomiting, and pain in the abdomen; the latter three require a doctor's immediate attention. More severe reactions, such as rashes (possibly including hives), breathing problems, and black stools or vomit, are not at all common; seek immediate treatment if they occur.
Diphenhydramine hydrochloride and acetaminophen	As directed on label.	Same comments as Diphenhydramine hydrochloride. Do not drink alcohol and use

Excedrine PM Caplets		products containing acetamino-phen. The combination can cause liver damage. Do not take with other pain-relieving substances.
Diphenhydramine hydrochloride and magnesium salicylate *Doan's PM*	As directed on label.	Same comments as Diphen-hydramine hydrochloride. The following warnings apply to magnesium salicylate: Do not take at the same time as tetracycline medications; allow at least an hour between these medications. Do not take if breastfeeding; avoid taking during pregnancy, or contact a physician before-hand; risk varies with product. Do not take if you have ulcers or bleeding problems; consult with a doctor if you have had ulcers or gout in the past, and if you have asthma or polyps in the nasal passages. Common side effects include indigestion, ringing in the ears, nausea, vomiting, and pain in the abdomen; the latter three require a doctor's immediate attention. More severe reac tions, such as rashes (possibly including hives), breathing problems, and black stools or vomit, are not at all common; seek immediate treatment if they occur.
Doxylamine succinate *Nytol Maximum Strength Caplets; Unisom*	As directed on label.	Same comments as Diphen-hydramine hydrochloride.

Some individuals develop a psychological dependence on sleep aids and continue to take them after they have outlived their usefulness. Avoid using these products often. Instead, try natural approaches.

NATURAL REMEDIES

If you suffer from insomnia, eat a dinner that is high in carbohydrates and contains little or no protein. Carbohydrates help to increase serotonin levels in the brain, which facilitate relaxation and sleep; protein blocks the process. Avoid stimulants, such as caffeine, and depressants, such as alcohol. Also, avoid eating sweet snacks before bedtime. Foods that are high in tryptophan, such as turkey, bananas, figs, dates, yogurt, tuna, whole bran crackers, and nut butter, are helpful to eat before sleeping.

Exercise and stress-management techniques (such as meditation and deep breathing) help many individuals overcome insomnia. So do soothing herbal teas, such as chamomile. The following table lists several natural supplements that encourage better sleep.

Natural Remedy	Dosage	Comments
Amantra	As directed on label.	A clinically proven natural herbal remedy for anxiety and sleep disorders that does not producing a morning "hangover" effect. The use of alcohol with this product may have an additive effect. Do not use this product and drive.

Kava kava	*For increased relaxation and reduced anxiety:* 45 to 70 mg of kavalactones (usually 1 capsule/ tablet), 3 times daily; *For assistance in falling asleep:* 180 to 210 mg of kavalactones	Do not take with alcohol. Use a product whose label states that it is standardized to known levels of kavalactones, so that each tablet or capsule provides 45 to 70 mg of kavalactones.
Melatonin *Melatonex; Knock-Out*	As directed on label.	Not recommended for long-term use. A hormone that naturally occurs in the body and serves as an antioxidant. It helps to regulate and aid sleep. Due to lack of sufficient long-term research at this time, melatonin is not recommended for pregnant and lactating women; individuals who have autoimmune diseases and immune system cancers; individuals who have signifi- cant allergies; and children (who already naturally produce considerable melatonin).
Valerian	150 to 300 mg, an hour before bedtime	Be sure to use a standardized extract that lists, on the label, that the active constituents are standardized to contain n0.8-percent valeric acid. Do not operate a vehicle while under the effects of this herb.

Jock Itch

This condition, also termed *tinea cruris*, usually occurs in males. It is caused by a wide variety of microorganisms. There is typically a ringed lesion that extends from the crotch area to the upper inner-thigh. Sometimes both thighs are affected. The scrotum is not usually involved, but may become acutely inflamed if candida (see page 118) is present. Recurrence is common with the fungi that cause jock itch, either due to microorganisms that continue to thrive on the skin or to reinfection.

There are several factors that put one at risk for jock itch. First, this condition is more common in the summer, due to the heat and the tendency to sweat. Second, tight clothing fosters the growth of the fungi responsible for jock itch. Finally, obesity is associated with the occurrence of jock itch. It may be difficult, in the early stages, to distinguish between jock itch and contact dermatitis, psoriasis, or candidiasis. If you have any question concerning the cause of the symptoms you are experiencing, see a dermatologist for an accurate diagnosis.

OTC REMEDIES

Treatment with a topical cream or lotion is usually effective for jock itch. Use an OTC at the first sign of this fungal growth. Always read the label before using any product.

OTC Remedy	Application	Comments
Aftate Spray Powder for Jock Itch	As directed on label.	Kills fungi. No common side effects. Further irritation of the skin due to use of this product is unusual.
Cruex Antifungal Powder/Spray Powder/Cream	As directed on label.	Same comments as *Aftate Spray Powder for Jock Itch.*
Desenex Precription Strength AF Cream/Spray Powder/Spray Liquid	As directed on label.	Same comments as *Aftate Spray Powder for Jock Itch.*
Lotrimin AF Antifungal Cream/Solution/ Lotion	As directed on label.	Same comments as *Aftate Spray Powder for Jock Itch.*
Tinactin Antifungal Jock Itch Cream/Spray Powder	As directed on label	Same comments as *Aftate Spray Powder for Jock Itch.*

NATURAL REMEDIES

In most cases, proper hygiene will help resolve jock itch. Wear loose clothing made of materials that "breathe," to allow air circulation to the affected area. Shower/bathe immediately after exercise and dry thoroughly. Try to wear absorbant material, such as cotton. The groin area should be separated from the scrotum by underwear.

In addition to keeping the area dry and clean, we still recommend the OTCs on the market. Also, keep in mind that recurring fungal infections can be indicative of depressed immunity. Be sure to follow a good multivitamin/mineral regimen to maintain healthy immune function. (See pages 14 to 20.)

Lactose Intolerance

Lactose is one of the sugars that is present in milk. The body breaks lactose down into its two component monosaccharides—glucose and galactose—through the use of an enzyme called *lactase*. This enzyme is released from the lining of the small intestine.

Lactose intolerance is the condition that results from the inability to digest lactose found in milk. People with this condition may get diarrhea from dairy products because the undigested lactose builds up and ferments in the feces. It is almost always caused by a deficiency in the enzyme lactase. In fact, lactose intolerance is extremely rare in people who are not deficient in lactase.

OTC REMEDIES

The following table lists several products on the market that can help prevent the symptoms of lactose intolerance. These remedies are supplements of lactase enzyme that help the body digest dairy. Always read the label carefully before using a product.

OTC Remedy	Dosage	Comments
LactAid Drops	As directed on label.	Several drops are added to milk, which is then shaken and refrigerated for 24 hours.
LactAid Caplets	As directed on label.	Available in original, extra, and ultra strengths. Take caplets with your first bite of dairy food. They act only on the food you are eating at the time, so take this remedy whenever you consume dairy foods.

NATURAL REMEDIES

The obvious and only true natural remedy for lactose intolerance is to avoid milk and all other dairy foods. The one exception is live-culture yogurt; the bacteria contained in this yogurt actually digest the lactose, as well as aid in other digestion processes. Also, some studies suggest that lactose intolerant individuals might absorb less calcium. Therefore, if you have this condition, consider supplementing with a good multi-vitamin/mineral and extra calcium so that you reach a daily calcium intake of 1,000 to 1,200 milligrams. Foods rich in calcium are another good option, a few of which are: broccoli; dried figs; spinach; tofu; and yogurt.

Leg Cramps

See Musclar Aches and Pains.

Lice

See Hair and Scalp Problems.

Lyme Disease

See Insect Bites.

Memory Loss

Decreased memory is often associated with aging. But memory loss is not natural to the aging process itself. Instead, it is a symptom of several disorders that simply become more likely to occur as we age. Memory loss is most frequently due to a decrease in circulation. This often happens as a result of atherosclerosis or "hardening of the arteries"—the loss of elasticity in the arterial walls and therefore the loss of their proper function, and/or the accumulation of plaques within the vessels. Atherosclerosis leads to reduced blood supply and, ultimately, the memory center in the brain does not receive adequate oxygen.

It is important to realize that temporary memory problems can occur at any age and are not a sure sign of serious illness. Nutrition plays a large role in memory capacity; nutrient deficiencies can certainly be responsible for memory loss. Also, stress, anxiety, and fatigue can affect memory. However, memory problems can be related to such conditions as Alzheimer's disease, hypothyroidism, hypoglycemia, chemical hypersensitivity, and exposure to heavy metals. So if the problem persists or worsens, consult a physician.

OTC REMEDIES

There are no OTC products for the enhancement of memory. However, there are several nutritional and herbal approaches that may combat memory loss. See "Natural Remedies," below.

NATURAL REMEDIES

A good approach to the prevention of memory loss is to follow the Five-A-Day Diet (page 21). It is important to consume adequate fruits and vegetables, which will provide you with proper nutrition. Also, practice stress-reduction techniques—for example, yoga, meditation, prayer, massage therapy. Be sure to exercise regularly. And most of all, use your brain! This is one of those "use it or lose it" situtations. It is critical to keep the brain active in order to maintain its abilities. Finally, several nutrients may be helpful in enhancing your memory health. See the following table for guidance.

Natural Remedy	Dosage	Comments
Ginkgo biloba *Bioginkg;* *Ginkogin;* *Ginkai;* *Ginkgomax;* *Ginkoba;* *Ginkgo Go*	As directed on label.	Increases circulation and, therefore, may improve memory. Some people experience a slight headache during the first few days of use. This side effect usually subsides within the first week.

Grape-seed extract or Pine bark extract *Pycnogenol*	25 to 50 mg, daily	Rich source of antioxidants. Grape-seed extract and pine bark extract are comparable substances.
Multivitamin/ mineral*	See pages 14 to 20.	See pages 14 to 20.
Vitamin C*	1,000 to 3,000 mg, daily	Safe for long-term maintenance.
Vitamin E*	400 IU, daily	Take with a meal. Antioxidant research has shown that this vitamin may be helpful in preventing memory loss. Mixed tocopherols supplying 400 IU of d-alpha tocopherol are preferred. Can be used for long-term maintenance.

* It is important that the discussed nutrients be part of a basic vitamin/mineral regimen so that the total daily amount of each nutrient obtained from both a multivitamin/mineral and other supplements is approximately the dosage indicated above.

Menopausal Problems

"The change of life," as menopause is sometimes called, indicates the cessation of ovulation in a woman and, therefore, the end of the child-bearing years. Menopause is a highly individual matter: it occurs earlier in some women than in others; it affects some more strongly than others; for some, menopause starts, then stops, and then starts up again. Menopause generally occurs around the age of fifty and can last for up to five years.

Hot flashes, dizziness, depression, breathing difficulties, heart palpitations, and vaginal dryness are common symptoms of menopause. It is believed that these symptoms may be caused by a decrease in estrogen production. (If a woman also suffers from hypoglycemia, these symptoms can be aggravated.) Estrogen replacement therapy (ERT) is the most common treatment for the symptoms of menopause. However, ERT poses some problems of its own—estrogen therapy can result in fluid retention and also may increase the severity and risk of heart problems, cancer, asthma, migraine, kidney stones, and epilepsy. Usually, taking the lowest possible dose of estrogen is the best choice. Treatment requires consultation with a doctor.

Many women simply opt to manage menopause naturally. It is smart to read as much as possible on the subject. In addition, there are various support and social groups that provide a forum for worries and frustrations. Such groups can be very helpful.

OTC REMEDIES

The products listed in the first section of the following table are analgesics—substances that relieve or reduce pain. They should alleviate some of the uncomfortable symptoms associated with menopause. If you have experienced side effects from any nonprescription pain relievers, do not take any of these remedies without consulting your doctor. Also included in the table is a recommendation for a topical moisturizing product. Always read the label before using any product.

OTC Remedy	Dosage	Comments
Oral Pain-Relieving Medications		
Acetaminophen *Excedrin Aspirin-Free; Panadol; Tylenol*	325 mg regular strength; generally, 500 mg extra strength	Do not drink alcohol and use products containing acetaminophen. The combination can cause liver damage. Do not take with other analgesics. Some products, such as *Tylenol*, are available in regular, junior, and extra strength.
Aspirin (acetylsalicylic acid) *Ascriptin; Bayer; Bufferin; Ecotrin; Empirin; Excedrin Extra Strength*	325 mg regular strength; generally, 500 mg extra strength	If pregnant, consult your doctor before taking products containing aspirin. Do not take products containing aspirin during the last three months of pregnancy. Children and teens should not use products containing aspirin for colds, flus, or chickenpox. Do not take products containing aspirin if you have asthma, stomach problems, gastric ulcers, bleeding problems, or if you are allergic to aspirin.
Ibuprofen *Advil; Arthritis Foundation Ibuprofen; Motrin IB; Nuprin*	200 mg	If pregnant, consult your doctor before taking this remedy. Do not take products containing this ingredient during the last three months of pregnancy. Do not take this ingredient if you are allergic to aspirin. Do not take this ingredient with any other analgesics. Consult your doctor before taking this remedy with prescription drugs.
Ketoprofen *Orudis KT*	12.5 mg	Same comments as Ibuprofen.

Naproxen sodium *Aleve*	220 mg	If pregnant, consult your doctor before taking this remedy. Do not take products containing this ingredient during the last three months of pregnancy. Do not take this ingredient with any other analgesics. Consult your doctor before taking this remedy with prescription drugs.

Topical Treatment for Vaginal Dryness

Gyne-Moistrin Vaginal Moisturizing Gel	As directed on label.	May remedy vaginal discomfort. Discontinue use if irritation occurs.

When used responsibly, acetaminophen, aspirin, ibuprofen, ketoprofen, and naproxen sodium are safe and effective. Look for single-ingredient products. If you have questions or concerns regarding the safety and effectiveness of any product, consult your doctor or pharmacist.

NATURAL REMEDIES

Regular exercise helps alleviate the symptoms of menopause, so make it a part of your routine. For example, several times a week, set aside a specific time to walk or to swim. As far as dietary factors are concerned, try to avoid dairy products. Also, soy protein contains phytoestrogens that may help balance hormones and relieve symptoms. Drinking a blended soy shake every morning will contribute to better well-being. For example, blend 2 heaping tablespoons of soy protein; 4 to 6 ounces of cranberry juice cocktail; 4 to 6 ounces of water (to taste); 1 heaping tablespoon of oat bran; 4 frozen strawberries; $\frac{1}{2}$ frozen banana; and 1 tablespoon of flaxseed oil.

There are several easy-to-find natural substances that ease the uncomfortable symptoms of menopause. See the table below. Alternative/complementary practitioners can suggest additional herbal, homeopathic, and other approaches.

Natural Remedy	Dosage	Comments
Bioflavonoids	500 mg, 3 times daily	Nutrients that serve many functions, some of which are the reduction of pain, maintenance of capillary health, and antibacterial action. Taken with 500 mg of vitamin C each time, they may help to relieve hot flashes.
Black cohosh extract	40 mg daily, in divided doses; for example, take 20 mg in the morning and 20 in the evening	May take up to 8 weeks to be fully effective in suppressing hot flashes. Since long-term usage is not well-documented, take a month off every six months. If you are on estrogen therapy, consult your physician before taking this herb.
Dong quai	As directed on label.	A traditional remedy used throughout Asia. Reports of effectiveness are anecdotal; there is little research on this herb.
Multivitamin/ mineral*	See pages 14 to 20.	See pages 14 to 20.
Promensil	1 tablet, daily	Take with meals. Use for a minimum of two months.

		A natural plant estrogen that may have a hormone-balancing effect.
Rejuvex	As directed on label.	A vitamin/mineral formula designed specifically for problems associated with menopause.
Vitamin C*	500 mg, 3 times daily	When taken with 500 mg of bioflavonoids, 3 times daily, may help to relieve hot flashes. Safe for long-term maintenance.
Vitamin E*	400 IU, daily	Take with a meal. Mixed tocopherols supplying 400 IU of d-alpha tocopherol are preferred. Can be used for long-term maintenance. Some women find this vitamin helpful in relieving menopause-related symptoms, but it may take up to three months to start helping.
Vitex (also called Agnus-castus; shaste tree; monk's pepper)	As directed on label.	This herb may help to balance hormones.

* It is important that the discussed nutrients be part of a basic vitamin/mineral regimen so that the total daily amount of each nutrient obtained from both a multivitamin/mineral and other supplements is approximately the dosage indicated above.

Migraine

See also Headache.

A migraine is a severe headache caused by extreme dilation or constriction of blood vessels in the brain. It is often accompanied by: visual symptoms, such as blurred vision; gastrointestinal disturbances, such as nausea and vomiting; and numbness and tingling in the limbs. The exact cause of migraine is unknown, but stress, constipation, allergies, and lack of exercise have been linked to this condition.

A short period of depression, restlessness, irritability, and lack of appetite may precede a migraine attack. It generally begins with a throbbing headache, which is frequently located behind or above one eye. In addition, "classic" migraine, as opposed to the "common" migraine, is accompanied by an aura—a disturbance of vision involving sparks and flashes or other patterns of light—as well as speech disturbance and weakness. Additional senses, particularly the sense of smell, may become distorted during a migraine.

An individual can experience a migraine at any age, but those who suffer from them usually start getting migraines between the ages of ten and thirty. Migraines are not uncommon; approximately 10 percent of the population experience them. This condition is far more frequent in women than in men. Furthermore, there is a family history of migraine in over 50 percent of cases.

OTC REMEDIES

The products listed in the following chart are analgesics—substances that relieve or reduce pain. If you have experienced side effects from any nonprescription pain relievers, do not take any of these remedies

without consulting your doctor. Always read the label
before using a product.

OTC Remedy	Dosage	Comments
Acetaminophen *Excedrin Aspirin-Free; Panadol; Tylenol*	325 mg regular strength; generally, 500 mg extra strength	Do not drink alcohol and use products containing acetamino-phen. The combination can cause liver damage. Do not take with other analgesics. Some products, such as *Tylenol*, are available in regular, junior, and extra strength.
Aspirin (acetylsalicylic acid) *Ascriptin Bayer; Bufferin; Ecotrin; Empirin; Excedrin Extra Strength*	325 mg regular strength; generally, 500 mg extra strength	If pregnant, consult your doctor before taking products containing aspirin. Do not take products containing aspirin during the last three months of pregnancy. Children and teens should not use products containing aspirin for colds, flus, or chickenpox. Do not take products contain-ing aspirin if you have asthma, stomach problems, gastric ulcers, bleeding problems, or if you are allergic to aspirin.
Ibuprofen *Advil; Arthritis Foundation Ibuprofen; Motrin IB; Nuprin*	200 mg	If pregnant, consult your doctor before taking this remedy. Do not take products containing this ingredient during the last three months of pregnancy. Do not take this ingredient if you are allergic to aspirin. Do not take this ingredient with any other analgesics. Consult your doctor before taking this remedy with prescription drugs.
Ketoprofen *Orudis KT*	12.5 mg	Same comments as Ibuprofen.

Naproxen sodium *Aleve*	220 mg	If pregnant, consult your doctor before taking this remedy. Do not take products containing this ingredient during the last three months of pregnancy. Do not take this ingredient with any other analgesics. Consult your doctor before taking this remedy with prescription drugs.

When used responsibly, acetaminophen, aspirin, ibuprofen, ketoprofen, and naproxen sodium are safe and effective. Look for single-ingredient products. If you have questions or concerns regarding the safety and effectiveness of any product, consult your doctor or pharmacist. It is important to note that some headache remedies contain ingredients that may aggravate your condition, such as caffeine.

NATURAL REMEDIES

In some cases, dietary changes can help prevent and treat migraines. Some people experience migraines as a result of food allergies, and can relieve them by avoiding problem foods. For more information on food allergies, see page 188. A nutritionally oriented doctor can help identify which foods are the culprits.

Salt appears to be a contributing factor for many migraine sufferers, as do dairy products. Also foods and beverages that can cause constriction or relaxation of blood vessels should be avoided—for example, caffeinated beverages; chocolate; and alcohol. Citrus fruits and acid-producing, fried, fatty, and greasy foods can also contribute to or trigger migraines. Other common migraine-causing substances include: foods that contain tyramine (for example, red wine; cheese); pesticides; additives; preservatives; eggs; peanuts; curry; and grains such as wheat. Eating plenty of whole, unprocessed foods may help. It is extremely important to include plenty of fresh fruits and vegetables in your diet. (See the Five-A-Day Diet, page 21.)

There are some very effective alternative approaches to treating migraines, including chiropractic, biofeedback, meditation, acupuncture, and acupressure. Undoubtedly, stress can cause migraines. Therefore, make an effort to identify and remove, as much as possible, the stressors in your life. In addition to the aforementioned techniques, regular exercise may help to reduce stress and enhance general health. Finally, the supplements listed in the following table may be helpful.

Natural Remedy	Dosage	Comments
Feverfew *Mygrafew*	125 mg, 2 times daily	To prevent migraine headaches, take this substance on a daily basis. Make sure the product contains at least 0.2-percent partheno-lide. Also, note the expiration date on the bottle. Partheno-lide is relatively unstable; the closer the product gets to the expiration date, the less likely there will be enough partheno-lide present for the product to be effective.

Ginkgo biloba	Up to 240 mg, daily	Use a standardized extract containing 24-percent ginkgoflavone glycosides and 6-percent terpene lactones. May be beneficial in preventing migraine due to its ability to inhibit platelet activating factor. Can cause minor headaches when initially taken. This effect subsides usually within the first week of use.
Kava kava	140 to 210 mg of kavalactones	Has a mellowing effect that may be helpful for the treatment of stress-related migraines.
Multivitamin/ mineral*	See pages 14 to 20.	See pages 14 to 20. Be sure this supplement supplies 400 mg of magnesium and a minimum of 400 mg of calcium; 1,000 mg or more daily of calcium may decrease the incidence of migraine.
Valerian	300 to 500 mg	Use a standardized extract. Has traditionally been used for relaxation at bedtime, but may be helpful in reducing the incidence of recurring headaches due to stress. Do not drive a vehicle while under the effects of this herb.
Vitamin B$_2$* (also called riboflavin)	400 mg, daily	Among other functions, this vitamin is important for energy production and for healthy eyes.
Vitamin D*	400 IU, daily	Some migraine sufferers get relief from 1,000 mg of calcium and 400 IU of vitamin D daily.

* It is important that the discussed nutrients be part of a basic vitamin/mineral regimen so that the total daily amount of each nutrient obtained from both a multivitamin/mineral and other supplements is approximately the dosage indicated above.

Mood Disorders

"Mood disorders" is a general category that includes anxiety and depression. These are, unfortunately, common problems for people of all ages in our society. Symptoms can include fatigue; nervousness (even panic); tremors; loss of excitement/energy; and despair. Prescription drugs used to treat the symptoms of these mood disorders are among the most lucrative products on the market. Common mood disorders can be linked to one or more factors, such as life circumstances, psychological problems, and dietary imbalances (such as excess alcohol, sugar, or caffeine). Some natural remedies may be useful in managing mild cases of anxiety or depression. If the problem persists or worsens, see a physician or therapist. Do not self-diagnose and self-treat any moderate to severe mood disorders.

OTC REMEDIES

There are no recommended OTC products for the treatment of anxiety and depression. However, some natural substances may be effective, as described in the following section below.

NATURAL REMEDIES

It is important to seek the advice and diagnosis of a doctor or therapist. He or she can design a regimen that may reduce the symptoms of your mood disorder. To help manage daily anxiety and depressive feelings, it is important to follow a healthy diet, such as the Five-A-Day Diet (see page 21). Make regular exercise a part of your routine, and practice stress-reduction techniques, such as yoga and meditation. Other alternative/complementary therapies, including massage and biofeedback, may also help. Finally, consider the supplements listed in the following table.

Natural Product	Dosage	Comments
For Minor Depression (which lasts less than two weeks)		
St. John's wort *Kira; Movanna; Centrum; Bayer*	125 to 250 mg, 3 times daily	Take with a meal. Until further research is done, do not take with MAO-inhibiting drugs, *Prozac*, or other antidepressant drugs. Use standardized extract products that contain 0.3-percent hypericin. If taking the brand *Kira*, take dose 1 to 3 times daily, with meals. See a physician if symptoms persist.
For Anxiety or Excessive Stress		
Amantra	As directed on label.	A clinically proven natural herbal remedy for anxiety and sleep disorders. If drowsiness occurs—especially likely with the nighttime dosage—take necessary precautions; do not drive. The use of alcohol with this product may have an additive effect.
Kava kava	200 mg, up to 3 times daily	Use standardized extract products that contain 30-percent kavalactones. Do not drink alcohol when using kava. The combination can cause drowsiness. Do not drive if drowsiness occurs.

Multivitamin/ mineral	See pages 14 to 20.	See pages 14 to 20. Be sure that your multivitamin/ mineral regimen includes 400 mg of magnesium daily.

Morning Sickness

See also Pregnancy-Related Problems.

This condition involves nausea and vomiting during early pregnancy. It is experienced by about half of all women who become pregnant. Although it is called "morning sickness," the difficulties associated with this condition can occur at any time of the day. It is important that the nausea and vomiting not keep a woman from eating or drinking. If morning sickness is severe and dehydration results from vomiting, hospitalization may be necessary. But usually, morning sickness is self-manageable.

OTC REMEDIES

The FDA has approved no drugs for the treatment of morning sickness. Fortunately, there are several natural substances that may bring relief from nausea and vomiting. See the following "Natural Remedies" section.

NATURAL REMEDIES

The most effective natural way to treat morning sickness and the resulting reduced appetite is to eat small meals throughout the day, rather than three regular-sized meals. Plain crackers and whole-wheat toast are helpful, as are bland foods such as bouillon soup, consomme, rice, and pasta. Eating before rising may prevent nausea; take an early morning cracker before getting out of bed.

Some women find that herbal teas are comforting. Suggested types of tea are peppermint, raspberry leaf, dried peachtree leaf, and chamomile. Also, taking ginger root or ginger powder can relieve the symptoms of this condition, as can several other natural remedies. See the table below for instructions. Keep in mind that any product that a woman takes for morning sickness affects the growing fetus.

Natural Remedy	Dosage	Comments
Ginger	*For standardized extracts:* as directed on label; *For capsules/tablets of powdered ginger:* 1 to 2 g daily, in divided doses— for example, take 500 mg, 2 to 4 times daily	Standard extracts are preferable.
Multivitamin/ mineral or prenatal vitamins	As directed on label.	Take with a meal. Be sure the supplement contains at least 50 mg of vitamin B_6. If not, take a separate supplement of vitamin B_6 with a meal. Be sure that the supplement contains at least 400 mg of magnesium. If not, an additional supplement should be taken. The supplement should also provide what is recognized as

the suitable amount of calcium during pregnancy—currently 1,200 to 1,500 mg daily. If it doesn't, an additional supplement should be taken.

Motion Sickness

Repetitive acceleration and deceleration at angles and in a straight line result in motion sickness. Such movement causes the sensory organs to send mixed signals to the brain, which then misinterprets them. The symptoms of this condition include severe headache, nausea, and vomiting. Various modes of movement can induce motion sickness, including the movement of the following: car; bus; train; boat; airplane; a swing; even travel in outer space! (Motion sickness in space travel is called space adaptation syndrome and is a major problem for astronauts during the first few days in space.) Motion sickness can also be initiated by visual stimuli, such as a moving horizon; by fumes, smoke, and carbon monoxide; by poor ventilation; and by emotional factors, such as fear or anxiety. It affects women more frequently than it does men. Interestingly, children under the age of two and the elderly rarely experience motion sickness.

OTC REMEDIES

The following table lists OTC products that help prevent and reduce motion sickness. Always read the label before using a product.

OTC Remedy	Dosage	Comments
Dimenhydrinate *Dramamine Liquid/Tablets*	As directed on label.	Available in regular tablets, chewable tablets, and liquid for children. Commonly causes drowsiness, dizziness, and dryness of the mouth, throat, and nasal passages. Take necessary precautions and maintain fluid intake. More severe side effects, such as vision changes, rashes, and difficulty urinating, are uncommon.
Meclizine hydrochloride *Bonine Chewable Tablets; Dramamine II*	As directed on label.	Commonly causes drowsiness. Take necessary precautions. Additional side effects, such as headache, digestive problems, mouth/throat/nasal dryness, and more severe reactions are uncommon.

If you have questions or concerns regarding the safety and effectiveness of any product, consult your doctor or pharmacist. Valid concerns have been expressed by authorities in the consumer-health field regarding the safety and effectiveness of products that contain certain chemicals. The following warning has been issued:

• Products containing only meclizine should be taken for limited use only.

NATURAL REMEDIES

It is easier to prevent motion sickness than to treat it. If a person is prone to motion sickness, then junk food, processed foods, alcohol, smoke, and food odors should all be avoided before and during the time of motion. If sailing, lie down with eyes closed at the first sign of sickness. If sitting in a car, focusing on a steady and distant object (such as the horizon line) may help to reduce nausea from the overstimulation of the quickly passing objects outside of the car. See the following table for more suggestions.

Natural Remedy	Dosage	Comments
Ginger	*Standardized extract:* as directed on label; *Powdered form:* 1 to 2 g in capsules/tablets, dividing the dose—for example, 500 mg, 2 to 4 times daily	Standardized extract is preferable. If possible, start taking ginger the day before departure.
Peppermint	*Tea:* as needed; *Lozenges:* as needed	Soothing to the stomach.

Muscular Aches and Pains

Aches and pains of the muscles are common among athletes, people who work out, and those who are out of shape but suddenly engage in a strenuous physical activity like the office softball game. If a muscle is pushed beyond its capability, it will "knot up" (remain contracted) because of strain; it will not relax after the activity ceases.

In a similar manner, ligaments, which connect bone to muscle, can become strained and cause pain.

Sometimes the ligaments may actually tear, resulting in a sprain. Sprains are often caused by twisting movements, hard falls, and sudden movements. Another common source of aches and pains is damage to the soft tissue around the joints in the back, knees, ankles, fingers, and wrists. When such tissue is injured and bruised, swelling and soreness result.

In contrast to the pain caused by the above-discussed injuries, muscle cramping is frequently a result of nutritional deficiency. Sometimes conditions such as arthritis, anemia, and poor circulation may cause muscle cramping. It can be caused by certain drugs as well—for example, diuretics. Most cramps occur at night. If muscle cramps occur during the day, see a doctor to rule out more serious causes of the cramping, such as drug toxicity or serious injury to the muscle. Also, see your physician if muscular pain is accompanied by a fever, if you are experiencing muscle spasms that are causing weakness, tingling, or numbness, or if spasms do not improve within thirty minutes.

OTC REMEDIES

The following table lists products that bring relief from muscular aches and pains. Those listed in the first section of the table are analgesics—substances that relieve or reduce pain. If you have experienced side effects from any nonprescription pain relievers, do not take any of these remedies without consulting your doctor. The products listed in the second section are to be applied directly to the sore area. Always read the label before using a product.

OTC Remedy	Application/Dosage	Comments
Oral Pain-Relieving Medications		
Acetaminophen *Excedrin Aspirin-Free; Panadol; Tylenol*	325 mg regular strength; generally, 500 mg extra strength	Do not drink alcohol and use products containing acetaminophen. The combination can cause liver damage. Do not take with other analgesics. Some of these products, such as *Tylenol,* are available in regular, junior, and extra strength.
Aspirin (acetylsalicylic acid) *Ascriptin; Bayer; Bufferin; Ecotrin; Empirin; Excedrin Extra Strength*	325 mg regular strength; generally, 500 mg extra strength	If pregnant, consult your doctor before taking products containing aspirin. Do not take products containing aspirin during the last three months of pregnancy. Children and teens should not use products containing aspirin for colds, flus, or chickenpox. Do not take products containing aspirin if you have asthma, stomach problems, gastric ulcers, bleeding problems, or if you are allergic to aspirin.
Ibuprofen *Advil; Arthritis Foundation Ibuprofen; Motrin IB; Nuprin*	200 mg	If pregnant, consult your doctor before taking this remedy. Do not take products containing this ingredient during the last three months of pregnancy. Do not take this ingredient if you are allergic to aspirin. Do not take this ingredient with any other analgesics. Consult your doctor before taking this remedy with prescription drugs.
Ketoprofen *Orudis KT*	12.5 mg	Same comments as Ibuprofen.

Magnesium salicylate *Doan's Regular Strength*	377 mg regular strength; generally, 580 mg extra strength	If pregnant, consult your doctor before taking this remedy. Do not take products containing this ingredient during the last three months of pregnancy. Do not take this ingredient with any other analgesics. Do not take if you are on a sodium-restricted regimen, or if you have peptic ulcers or any bleeding conditions. Common side effects include nausea, vomiting, and pain in the abdomen; seek medical help immediately. Other common effects, though less harmful and not requiring immediate attention, include indigestion/heartburn and ringing in the ears.
Naproxen sodium *Aleve*	220 mg	If pregnant, consult your doctor before taking this remedy. Do not take products containing this ingredient during the last three months of pregnancy. Do not take this ingredient with any other analgesics. Consult your doctor before taking this remedy with prescription drugs.
Topical Products		
Bengay Ointment/Cream	As directed on label.	Also available in a greaseless cream. Temporarily reduces pain.
Capsaicin *Capzasin-P Analgesic Creme*	As directed on label.	Temporarily reduces pain.

When used responsibly, acetaminophen, aspirin, ibuprofen, ketoprofen, magnesium salicylate, and naproxen sodium are safe and effective. Look for single-ingredient products. If you have questions or concerns regarding the safety and effectiveness of any product, consult your doctor or pharmacist.

NATURAL REMEDIES

Massage and regular exercise are good ways to prevent and/or treat muscle aches and pains. Stretching should become a routine part of your lifestyle. For leg cramps, increase the amount of potassium-rich foods in your diet, such as bananas and dried fruits. Plenty of fruits and vegetables is important for physical health; we recommend the Five-A-Day Diet (see page 21). Also, add the appropriate nutrients listed in the table below.

Natural Remedy	Dosage	Comments
For Muscle Aches and Pains, Including Leg Cramps		
Calcium*	Minimum of 1,000 mg, daily	Take with a meal. Involved in regulating the contraction and relaxation of muscles.
Multivitamin/ mineral*	See pages 14 to 20.	See pages 14 to 20.
Vitamin E*	400 IU, daily	Take with a meal. Mixed tocopherols supplying 400 IU of d-alpha tocopherol are preferred. Can be used for long-term maintenance.

Magnesium*	400 mg, daily	Take with a meal. Mineral involved in muscle relaxation. Deficiency can cause muscle spasms, tremors, convulsions.
For Leg Cramps Due to Poor Circulation		
Ginkgo biloba *Bioginkgo;* *Ginkogin;* *Ginkai;* *Ginkgomax;* *Ginkoba;* *Ginkgo Go*	40 mg, 3 times daily, or 60 mg, 2 times daily	Make sure that product is standardized to 24-percent flavonglycosides. Maximum effect takes between 4 and 6 weeks. Some people experience a slight headache during the first few days of use. This usually disappears within the first week.
For Other Leg Conditions That Appear to Be Muscular But Are Really Vascular (such as a feeling of "heavy legs")		
Horse chestnut extract *Venostat*	1 tablet (approximately 17 to 35 mg) every 12 hours, with water, for 4 to 6 weeks, providing a total daily dose of 35 to 70 mg, daily	If taking a generic product, make sure that the product is standardized to 16- to 21-percent Escin (sometimes spelled Aescin). Will help to strengthen the vasculature and prevent fluids from leaking out of the vessels and into the leg tissues.

* It is important that the discussed nutrients be part of a basic vitamin/mineral regimen so that the total daily amount of each nutrient obtained from both a multivitamin/mineral and other supplements is approximately the dosage indicated above.

Nail Problems

The nails, which protect the sensitive fingertips and toetips, are made of protein, keratin, and sulfur. Nail problems are frequently caused by nutritional deficiencies and can result in many abnormalities. For example, hangnails are associated with a lack of vitamin C and folic acid. Lack of adequate protein also plays a role in hangnail formation. Dry, brittle nails can result from insufficient amounts of calcium and vitamin A. Horizontal and vertical ridges in the nails indicate a lack of B vitamins and/or iron deficiency. In addition, if the body does not have enough hydrochloric acid, nail splitting may occur. And fungus may form under and around the nails if there is a lack of lactobacillus in the body.

Covering up nail problems with cosmetics may also cover up health problems that need to be addressed. Problems with the nails are often symptomatic of disorders in other parts of the body. Nail changes may indicate serious illness, such as heart problems, a liver or kidney disorder, rheumatoid arthritis, thyroid problems, hormonal imbalances, or cirrhosis of the liver. See a nutritionist or a naturopathic physician if you notice changes in the texture and health of your nails. These professionals can offer helpful dietary advice, as well as information on possible disorders that are causing the problem.

OTC REMEDIES

If you have fungus around the nails, a helpful active ingredient is terbinafine 1%. It can be found in *Lamisil* cream. This product may provide a faster cure than other OTC antifungals used for athlete's foot, jock itch, and ringworm.

NATURAL REMEDIES

Nail health can be enhanced by following several natural approaches. First, when caring for your nails, avoid cutting the cuticles. Use a base coat when applying nail polish. Wear cotton-lined gloves when doing housework. As for dietary advice, a high-protein diet rich in vegetables and fruits will help. Furthermore, minor nail problems can sometimes be corrected by taking a multivitamin/mineral in addition to vitamin A daily. See the following table for supplementation instructions on these and other natural products that can be helpful.

Natural Remedy	Dosage	Comments
Hydrolyzed gelatin Knox Gelatin; Knox NutraJoint; Arthred G	*For Knox Gelatin products:* 1 tsp, daily, mixed into favorite beverage; *For Arthred G:* 2 tsp, daily, mixed into favorite beverage	Contains a proprietary hydrolyzed gelatin that may enhance nail health and, at the same time, help to maintain healthy joints.
Multivitamin/ mineral*	See pages 14 to 20.	See pages 14 to 20. Be sure that your multivitamin/ mineral regimen includes 1,200 mg of calcium, daily. If not, take an additional calcium supplement.
Vitamin A*	10,000 to 25,000 IU, daily	Take with a meal. 10,000 IU is safe for long-term maintenance; higher doses should not be taken for longer than 14 days. This vitamin can be toxic when taken in large amounts for a long period of time.

* It is important that the discussed nutrients be part of a basic vitamin/mineral regimen so that the total daily amount of each nutrient obtained from both a multivitamin/mineral and other supplements is approximately the dosage indicated above.

Obesity

This condition is characterized by the excessive accumulation of body fat. A body weight 20-percent higher than that listed in standard height-weight tables is considered (arbitrarily, some may say) as obesity. Current estimates are that 24 percent of men and 27 percent of women are obese. The incidence of obesity varies greatly with age, socioeconomic status, and race.

It is quite clear that, for many people, obesity results from consuming more calories than they expend. But at least seven major factors contribute to obesity: genetic factors; social factors; endocrine and metabolic factors; psychological factors; poor diet; levels of physical activity, and eating disorders. However the factors influence the condition, the bottom line is that obesity is associated with high blood pressure, kidney problems, liver disease, diabetes, pregnancy complications, and psychological problems.

The best way to lose weight is to develop a weight loss/control plan with your doctor or with a nutritionist that will help over the long-term. Short-term use of certain drugs may or may not be part of the plan. Mild obesity—the most common form, affecting over 90 percent of obese persons—can usually be handled by lifestyle changes, such as increased physical activity. Moderate obesity can be treated with changes in diet and with behavior therapy. Severe obesity (weight 100 percent or more over the accepted standard weight) may require surgery and severe changes to lifestyle regimens.

OTC REMEDIES

OTCs for weight loss are generally not recommended by physicians because these products are usually ineffective for long-term weight loss and may be harmful if used for long periods of time. However, there are a number of OTC items on the market. The following table lists just a couple of the major brands. Always read the label before using a product.

OTC Remedy	Dosage	Comments
Acutrim Tablets	As directed on label.	Do not take with asthma, allergy, and cough/cold medicines without consulting a physician. No common side effects. Occasionally, individuals experience dizziness, nausea, oral/nasal dryness, nervousness, insomnia, and minor headaches.
Dexatrim Caplets/Tablets	As directed on label.	Same comments as above.

NATURAL REMEDIES

As most people who have ever tried to shed a few pounds know, crash diets do not work. What does work is an overall program that focuses on improving lifestyle. Regular exercise should become a part of your daily routine. Improvements should be made to your diet, including the elimination of excess sugar and junk food and the addition of whole, pure foods. Eat a diet rich in vegetables and fruit. The Five-A-Day Diet (see page 21) is an example of a healthy approach to eating. Another tactic in controlling weight is to avoid foods that elevate blood sugar too quickly or to an excessive level. These foods include: white bread; puffed wheat; white flour; whole meal bread; spaghetti; and white rice.

In addition to the above-discussed recommendations, it is essential to drink plenty of water—six to eight glasses per day. Avoid animal fat, which contains a lot of the "bad" fats, and salt, which retains fluid and adds to bloating. Also, the consumption of fiber is critical to healthy digestion and excretion, which, in turn, is central to proper weight control. Caffeine can speed up metabolism and help burn fat. However, abuse of this substance can lead to many problems, including heart palpitations, anxiety, digestive ailments, etc. Caffeine is addictive and should not be relied upon. Ephedrine, described in the table below, is similar.

Stress management is very important when combatting obesity. Stress can eaily lead to overeating and can also impair the body's ability to burn fat. Try several stress-reduction techniques—yoga, meditation, massage—and see what works best for you. Finally, there are a number of natural substances that may help to resolve obesity problems. These are listed in the following table.

Natural Remedy	Dosage	Comments
Chitosan	As directed on label.	A fiber product made from the shells of shellfish. May block small amounts of fat from being absorbed.
Chromium picolinate	200 to 800 mcg, daily	May help control sugar cravings and regulate blood sugar. Chromium is a mineral, and picolinate is an amino acid that enables the body to employ chromium more efficiently.
Ephedrine	As directed on label.	From the herb *ephedra* or *ma huang*. Ephedrine can speed up metabolism and help burn fat. Note that this substance can raise blood pressure and should not be used by those who have elevated blood pressure. Check with a medical doctor before using this herbal substance. Ephedrine has been known to cause extreme health problems when abused, including fatality.
Guar gum	Found in some weight loss products.	Can contribute to a feeling of fullness, but may cause gas.
Pectin gum	Found in some weight loss products.	Can contribute to a feeling of fullness, but may cause gas.
Psyllium *Metamucil*	As directed on label.	A fiber that can give a feeling of fullness and acts as a mild laxative, as well.
Pyruvate	As directed on label.	Take with a meal. Nutrient shown to be helpful in weight loss, but only in relatively large doses, such as 2,000 to 5,000 mg daily, taken with meals.

Sequester	As directed on label.	A nutrient that may block small amounts of fat from being absorbed.

Oily Skin

See Skin Problems.

Osteoporosis

See also Menopausal Problems.

This condition is characterized by a generalized, progressive loss of bone-tissue mass and results in skeletal weakness. Bone fractures are common in people with osteoporosis, as are height loss, hip and back pain, and curvature of the spine. One of the major causes of this condition is a lack of calcium.

Osteoporosis primarily affects women and the risk of developing this condition increases with age. About one in four postmenopausal women have osteoporosis; estrogen deficiency is the leading cause among this population. To put statistics in perspective, about 15 to 20 million American women are affected by osteoporosis. Other causes of this condition include: inability to absorb calcium; lactose intolerance (see page 238); and insufficient amounts of both adrenal and ovarian hormones, including progesterone and DHEA (dehydroephiandrosterone).

Yet another cause of osteoporosis is too little weight-bearing exercise such as walking. Also, deficiencies in vitamins and minerals other than calcium can lead to this condition. It is important to consume adequate amounts of boron, copper, magnesium, manganese, zinc, and vitamins B_6, C, D, and K for proper bone metabolism. And sometimes it is not the insufficient consumption of vitamins and minerals that leads to osteoporosis, but the insufficient absorption by the gastrointestinal system. In addition, the excretion of calcium through the urine—caused by smoking, excessive consumption of alcohol, or foods high in protein, fat, sugar, or phosphorus—can contribute to this condition. Hyperparathyroidism is a treatable condition that also may cause osteoporosis. It is indicated by an increased serum-calcium level. Consult your doctor if a blood test shows that you have this problem.

A healthy diet provides for both the prevention and treatment of osteoporosis. Furthermore, some studies have indicated that after menopause, women who take natural progesterone, regardless of whether or not they take estrogen, have experienced improvement in bone density. Speak to your doctor about what kind of therapy would be most effective for you.

OTC REMEDIES

There are no "magic bullet" OTCs that can prevent or treat osteoporosis. The best approach is to follow the advice offered in the following "Natural Remedies" section. But there are products on the market that could give you a healthy dose of calcium, among which is *Tums 500 Calcium Supplement*. Always read the label before using a product, and follow your doctor's or nutritionist's advice concerning how much calcium you, as an individual, need to supplement.

NATURAL REMEDIES

To prevent osteoporosis, develop a regular exercise program for yourself that involves weight-bearing exercise. Also, a nutritionist can help you devise a diet that will provide you with proper nutrition. Your diet should be rich in whole foods and low-fat milk products that contain adequate amounts of protein.

For proper bone metabolism, be sure that you consume enough calcium, boron, copper, magnesium, manganese, zinc, and vitamins B_6, C, D, and K. These are often available through a good multivitamin/mineral regimen, but the ones detailed in the table below may require extra supplementation.

Natural Remedy	Dosage	Comments
Calcium*	*For premenopausal women:* 1,000 mg, daily; *For postmenopausal women:* 1,200 to 1,500 mg, daily	If your multivitamin/mineral regimen does not provide the proper dosage, take additional calcium supplements.
Magnesium*	400 to 800 mg, daily	If your multivitamin/mineral regimen does not provide the proper dosage, take additional magnesium supplements.
Manganese*	10 to 20 mg, daily	If your multivitamin/mineral regimen does not provide the proper dosage, take additional manganese supplements.

Multivitamin/ mineral,* including calcium *Centrum; Theragran M Tablets*	See pages xxx to xxx.	See pages xxx to xxx. Many supplement products are available in several formulas. For example, *Centrum* is available in regular, *Jr.,* and *Silver Formula for Adults 50+.*

* It is important that the discussed nutrients be part of a basic vitamin/mineral regimen so that the total daily amount of each nutrient obtained from both a multivitamin/mineral and other supplements is approximately the dosage indicated above.

PMS

See Premenstrual Syndrome.

Poison Ivy, Oak, Sumac

"Leaflets three, let it be!" is a handy childhood rhyme that will keep you at a safe distance from poison ivy. This common plant grows in many regions of the United States and causes hundreds of thousands of skin-poisoning cases each year. In addition to poison ivy, oak-leaf poison ivy, western poison oak, and poison sumac must be avoided. These latter poisonous plants are not three-leaved. Keep in mind that there are about sixty varieties of poisonous plants in the United States. It is important to take precautions during outdoor activities. If you and your family enjoy the outdoors, take some time to familiarize yourselves with the common poisonous plants in your area.

The symptoms of skin poisoning due to poison ivy, poison oak, and poison sumac usually appear within a few hours of contact, although it sometimes takes several days to feel the effects. A burning and itching sensation comes first, followed by redness, swelling, blistering, and a rash. Scratching the affected area can spread the irritation.

Anyone who plans to be out in nature should prevent exposure to these plants by wearing the proper protective clothing. Also be aware that clothing that comes into contact with such plants must be cleaned, as it carries the irritating substances and can cause a reaction to occur or recur. If you have come into contact with a poisonous plant, wash immediately or as soon as possible. Follow up with an OTC or natural remedy. See a doctor if you run a fever or if a widespread rash occurs on the eyes, mouth, or genitals.

OTC REMEDIES

The following table lists OTC products that relieve the symptoms of poison ivy and similar inflammations. Always read the label before using a product.

OTC Remedy	Application	Comments
Benadryl Itch Relief Cream/Spray/Gel	Apply to affected area, as directed on label.	Also available in children's and maximum-strength formulas. Reduces inflammation. Further skin irritation due to use of this product is uncommon.
Caladryl Lotion/Cream	Apply to affected area, as directed on label.	Also available in a cream for children.

Caldecort Cream/Spray	Apply to affected area, as directed on label.	Also available in *Light Cream*. Reduces inflammation. Further skin irritation due to use of this product is uncommon. Do not use if you are allergic to any cortisone products.
Cortaid Cream/ Ointment/ Spray	Apply to affected area, as directed on label.	The regular- and maximum-strength formulas are available in cream and ointment forms, while the maximum-strength formula is also available in spray form. Reduces inflammation. Further skin irritation due to use of this product is uncommon. Do not use if you are allergic to any cortisone products.
Cortizone for Kids Anti-Itch Creme	Apply to affected area, as directed on label.	Reduces inflammation. No common side effects. Further skin irritation due to use of this product is uncommon. Do not use if you are allergic to any cortisone products.
Cortizone-5 Creme/Ointment	Apply to affected area, as directed on label.	Same comments as *Cortizone for Kids Anti-Itch Creme*.
Coritzone-10 Creme/Ointment	Apply to affected area, as directed on label.	Same comments as *Cortizone for Kids Anti-Itch Creme*.
Ivy Block	Apply before contact with plants, as directed on label.	A protectant against poison oak and poison ivy. Apply to parts of the body that are likely to come into contact with these plants.
Technu	Apply after contact with plants, as directed on label.	Removes toxins. Use as soon as irritation begins, or even if you suspect you have come into contact with poisonous plants.

NATURAL REMEDIES

To relieve the skin reaction that comes from a poisonous plant, you can apply very hot, water-soaked compresses to the affected area for short periods of time. If you are not satisfied with using just a plain water-compress, try soaking the compress in diluted Burrow's solution (available in most drug stores). Also soothing to irritated skin is cool-water colloidal oatmeal soaks. Colloidal oatmeal is widely available in drug stores; the *Aveeno* brand is well-known.

If itching occurs, a paste made from water and any of the following may prove helpful: cornstarch; baking soda; oatmeal; or Epsom salts. To make this paste, mix 1 teaspoon of water with 3 teaspoons of the dry ingredient. Another option is to apply pure aloe vera juice/gel to the affected area to relieve itchiness or burning. Other helpful topical natural remedies include watermelon rind, tofu, and buttermilk mixed with sea salt (1 tablespoon of the salt to every pint of the buttermilk).

Poisoning

Poisoning is the most common cause of nonfatal accidents in the home. It is critically important that the phone numbers for the nearest Poison Control Center and emergency room are readily available at all times. The most common serious poisonings in children are from acetaminophen; aspirin; caustics, such as cleansing agents; iron; and hydrocarbons from such substances as paint thinners. Frequent culprits are common household chemicals stored under the kitchen sink, in the basement, and in the garage—drain and toilet bowl cleaners, dishwashing detergents, paints and paint products, gasoline, and petroleum products. Liquid products are much more dangerous than solids because greater amounts can be consumed before burning and other warning signals are sensed.

Prevention is paramount with poisoning. If poisoning does occur, call the Poison Control Center immediately. Often they will instruct you to empty the stomach right away by using syrup of ipecac. However, some cases are unique, so don't take measures until you have spoken with a trained representative. It may also be necessary to go to the nearest emergency room. If children are home alone, make sure they know who to call and what to do in case of poisoning.

OTC REMEDIES

The following table lists several OTC products that can be life-saving in the case of a poisoning emergency. Upon purchasing a product, familiarize yourself with the instructions for its use. Thus, if you must use it in an emergency, you will already know the drill. Be sure that you phone the Poison Control Center immediately upon suspicion of poisoning; unless you are trained in this area, do not make decisions on your own to take certain remedies. Keep these and all OTCs, along with other dangerous products, out of the reach of children.

OTC Remedy	Dosage	Comments
Charcoaid	As directed on label.	Available in original and *Charcoaid 2000*. Induces vomiting.
Ipecac Syrup	As directed on label.	Induces vomiting.

NATURAL REMEDIES

There are no recommended natural remedies for a poisoning situation. It is simply best to keep the above-suggested products in your medicine chest in case of an emergency, and to call a poison center or a physician immediately.

Pregnancy-Related Problems

See also Morning Sickness; Stretch Marks.

Many problems can occur during pregnancy. Some are simple and easily resolved, while others can be serious, even life-threatening. Among the most common problems that pregnant women experience are: backache; bleeding gums; constipation; dizziness; gas or flatulence; groin spasm or "stitches"; heartburn; hemorrhoids; insomnia; leg cramps; miscarriage or spontaneous abortion; mood changes; morning sickness; nasal congestion; nosebleeds; sciatica; skin problems; soreness; stretch marks; sweating; swelling of the hands and feet; varicose veins; and weight gain.

Whatever the problem, before a pregnant woman takes any prescription medication, over-the-counter drug, or nutritional supplement, or even if she simply experiences any of the symptoms given above, it is important to consult a doctor. The following should definitely be avoided during pregnancy: *Accutane;* alcohol; *Alka-seltzer;* antibiotics (for example, ampicillin, tetracycline); antihistamines; aspartame; aspirin; caffeine; cold pills; cough medicine; *Datril;* decongestants; *Di-Gel; Dilantin;* estrogens; *Gelusil; Maalox;* mineral oils; *Pepto-Bismol;* phenylalanine; *Rolaids; Tegison; Tums;* and *Tylenol.*

OTC REMEDIES

Unless otherwise directed by your physician, it is best to avoid OTC products and to follow natural remedies when it comes to treating conditions during pregnancy. But *any* form of treatment should be discussed with your health-care professional before use.

NATURAL REMEDIES

There are a number of ways to naturally manage common pregnancy-related problems. First, bleeding gums is a common symptom of pregnancy. Brushing your teeth three to four times daily, and flossing as well, will help prevent this problem. Also, ensure that your diet contains enough calcium, complete proteins, and vitamin C, all of which promote healthy tissue function and strengthen collagen. An increased intake of vitamin C will also reduce the incidence of nosebleeds and nasal congestion, as will eating fewer dairy products.

To decrease soreness in the rib area, change your position frequently. The movement will prevent stiffness and allow for better circulation. Similarly, for backache, avoid staying in one position for long periods of time. Do not wear high-heeled shoes. Furthermore, avoid forward bending and strong upward stretching. It is a good idea to make two to three minutes of careful stretching part of your daily routine.

Some pregnant women suffer from sciatica. This condition is characterized by pain, burning, tingling, or general discomfort anywhere along the sciatic nerve, which runs from the lower back down through the buttocks and legs. Physical therapists and chiropractors can offer effective treatment through massage therapy.

To relieve leg cramps, eat foods containing calcium and potassium, such as bananas, grapefruits, oranges, cottage cheese, yogurt, salmon, soybeans, almonds, and sesame seeds. Calcium and potassium are necessary for proper muscle function. Also, elevate your legs so that they are higher than your heart. Avoid standing in one place for too long. Walking will help to get the blood flowing.

To avoid dizziness, avoid changing positions quickly. Also, to prevent groin spasm, stitch, or pressure, daily exercise is helpful, but check first with a doctor. And when you are experiencing a spasm, breathe deeply, bend into the painful area, and rest on one side in bed until the spasm subsides.

Gastrointestinal problems often accompany pregnancy. To ease morning sickness, eat small, frequent meals and snack on whole grain crackers with nut butters or cheese. The herb ginger is effective in preventing vomiting. There are several options available for taking ginger: a cup of ginger tea; a powdered-ginger capsule; or two to five drops of ginger liquid tincture.

Be sure to add fresh and dried fruits to your diet if you experience constipation. In addition, make walking a part of your daily routine. To lessen gas, eat four to six small meals a day, instead of three big meals. Here too, walking is helpful. Eating smaller and more frequent meals and remaining physically active will also reduce heartburn.

To treat hemorrhoids, eat more roughage—raw vegetables and fruits—and elevate your feet and legs while defecating. Cold witch-hazel compresses applied to the affected area are soothing. And again, walking helps to better regulate your gastrointestinal system, thus reducing related problems.

Some women get insomnia during pregnancy—they cannot attain a good night's sleep. If you find yourself unable to rest well, increase your intake of foods rich in vitamin B. These foods will also help to reduce mood swings. Herbal teas containing chamomile, marjoram, or lemon balm induce relaxation. In addition, make the last meal of the day a high-carbohydrate, low-protein meal, to increase brain serotonin levels and encourage sleep onset. You may also want to try relaxation and meditation techniques, such as progressive muscle relaxation or transcendental meditation.

Stretch marks are a common condition for pregnant women. They are lines of discoloration on the skin, initially red and ultimately white, that result from the stretching caused by rapid weight gain. While stretch marks are permanent, they tend to fade quite well over time. A combination of virgin olive oil, aloe vera gel, vitamin E oil, and vitamin A oil applied to areas where marks commonly appear can be very helpful in preventing these marks.

Many pregnant women find that their hands and feet swell. It is important to consult your doctor if you experience swelling, as this could be a sign of a more severe condition. But for most women, swelling occurs simply as the result of fluid retention and hormonal changes. It can be lessened by avoiding highly processed foods, by wearing loose and comfortable clothing, and by walking. To prevent varicose veins, sit with your feet up higher than your heart and change positions frequently. Do not sit cross-legged and do not wear tight knee-socks, garters, belts, or high-heeled shoes. Support hose help to maintain proper circulation.

Some women get skin problems during pregnancy. If you find that you are breaking out in blemishes, do not wear make-up. It is critically important to maintain a balanced vitamin/mineral regimen, as well. And drink plenty of water, to keep your body cleansed and your skin hydrated.

During pregnancy, dress in loose, light clothing. This will allow you to feel more comfortable and to avoid sweating. Also avoid hot baths, as they will leave you feeling overheated. For more information on the discussed symptoms, please see the individual sections on the following: back pain; congestion, constipation; gas; hemorrhoids; insomnia; muscle aches and pains; mood disorders; morning sickness; skin problems; stretch marks; varicose veins; and weight gain.

Premenstrual Syndrome (PMS)

Premenstrual syndrome, often referred to as PMS, usually occurs approximately ten days before menstruation and subsides within hours of the onset of menstrual blood flow. This condition seems to be related to fluctuations in estrogen and progesterone levels in the body. Common symptoms of PMS are: nervousness; irritability; and emotional instability, including depression. Headaches, backaches, breast pain and tenderness, and bloated abdomen are also frequent symptoms.

The majority of women experience PMS symptoms, but the discomforts generally last for short periods of time and do not interfere with everyday living. However, some women experience symptoms that do disturb their daily functioning for hours or even days. Emotional outbursts of anger, suicidal thoughts, and violence can accompany PMS. In such cases, it is important to consult a doctor and discuss various forms of treatment.

OTC REMEDIES

The products listed in the following chart are analgesics—substances that relieve or reduce pain. If you have experienced side effects from any nonprescription pain relievers, do not take any of these remedies without consulting your doctor. Always read the label before using a product.

OTC Remedy	Dosage	Comments
For Menstrual Pain		
Acetaminophen *Excedrin Aspirin-Free; Panadol; Tylenol*	325 mg regular strength; generally, 500 mg extra strength	Do not drink alcohol and use products containing acetaminophen. The combination can cause liver damage. Do not take with other analgesics. Some of these products, such as *Tylenol,* are available in regular, junior, and extra strength.
Aspirin (acetylsalicylic acid) *Ascriptin, Bayer; Bufferin; Ecotrin; Empirin; Excedrin Extra Strength*	325 mg regular strength; generally, 500 mg extra strength	If pregnant, consult your doctor before taking products containing aspirin. Do not take products containing aspirin during the last three months of pregnancy. Children and teens should not use products containing aspirin for colds, flus, or chickenpox. Do not take products containing aspirin if you have asthma, stomach problems; gastric ulcers, bleeding problems, or if you are allergic to aspirin.
Ibuprofen *Advil; Arthritis Foundation Ibuprofen; Motrin IB; Nuprin*	200 mg	If pregnant, consult your doctor before taking this remedy. Do not take products containing this ingredient during the last three months of pregnancy. Do not take this ingredient if you are allergic to aspirin. Do not take this ingredient with any other analgesics. Consult your doctor before taking this remedy with prescription drugs.

Ketoprofen *Orudis KT*	12.5 mg	Same comments as Ibuprofen.
Naproxen sodium *Aleve*	220 mg	If pregnant, consult your doctor before taking this remedy. Do not take products containing this ingredient during the last three months of pregnancy. Do not take this ingredient with any other analgesics. Consult your doctor before taking this remedy with prescription drugs.

For Menstrual Pain and Other PMS Symptoms

Acetaminophen, caffeine, and pyrilamine maleate *Midol Maximum Strength Multi-Symptom Formula*	As directed on label.	Same comments as Acetaminophen.
Acetaminophen and pamabrom *Midol Teenage Multi-Symptom Formula*	As directed on label.	Same commments as Acetaminophen.
Acetaminophen, pamabrom, and pyrilamine maleate *Midol PMS Multi-Symptom Formula*	As directed on label.	Same comments as Acetaminophen.

When used responsibly, acetaminophen, aspirin, ibuprofen, ketoprofen, naproxen sodium, and the ingredients used in combination with them in the above-mentioned products are safe and effective. If you have questions or concerns regarding the safety and effectiveness of any product, consult your doctor or pharmacist.

NATURAL REMEDIES

To help relieve or reduce your symptoms of premenstrual syndrome, avoid the following substances: alcohol; caffeine; dairy products; processed, junk, or fast foods; red meat; salt; and sugar. In addition, do not smoke. The daily supplement regimen that is suggested in the following table is very helpful. And make time in your day for physical activity, as well as adequate rest. These lifestyle decisions will enhance your general well-being and make PMS more manageable.

Natural Remedy	Dosage	Comments
Black cohosh extract	40 mg, daily, in divided doses— for example, 20 mg in the morning, and 20 mg in the evening	May help to balance hormones; relieves menstrual cramps and associated back pain. May take up to two months for full effect to take place. Since long-term usage is not well-documented, take one month off after every six months of use. Do not use this herb during pregnancy or lactation. If you are on estrogen therapy, consult your physician before taking this herb.
Bromelain	As directed on label.	Relieves menstrual cramps.
Dandelion	As directed on label.	Reduces water retention.
Magnesium*	400 mg, daily	Important for muscle relaxation. Extra supplementation is needed only if this dose is not included in your multivitamin/mineral.

Multivitamin/ Mineral*	See pages 14 to 20.	See pages 14 to 20.
Siberian ginseng (*Eleutherococcus senticosus*)	100 to 200 mg, daily	Use standardized extract. Has a strengthening and stimulating effect, helping the body to adapt to change. Safe for long-term maintenance, but do not use this herb if you have high blood pressure, hypoglycemia, or heart problems. Can increase to 600 mg daily during the most troublesome time of the month.
Vitamin B$_6$*	50 mg, daily	Necessary for serotonin production. Serotonin deficiencies are linked to depression. Extra supplementation is needed only if this dose is not included in your multivitamin/ mineral.
Vitex (also called Agnus-castus; shaste tree, and monk's pepper)	As directed on the label.	Be sure to purchase a standardized extract. Take for at least four months, to determine if it is going to be effective.

* It is important that the discussed nutrients be part of a basic vitamin/mineral regimen so that the total daily amount of each nutrient obtained from both a multivitamin/mineral and other supplements is approximately the dosage indicated above.

Prostate Problems

The prostate, found in males, is a small gland that lies below the bladder and surrounds the urethra. It secretes fluids that increase sperm motility and fight infection. Prostate problems are receiving a great deal of attention today. Enlargement of the prostate (benign

prostatic hypertrophy, or BPH) occurs in 40 to 60 percent of men over the age of forty, as hormones shift during the aging process. When enlarged, the prostate can
block the flow of urine and/or cause other urinary tract
problems, such as difficulty urinating and nighttime
awakening to urinate. If you have these symptoms,
suspect prostate problems and consult a physician for
an accurate diagnosis; do not self-diagnose.

OTC REMEDIES

There are no OTC remedies that restore prostate
health. However, see the following "Natural Remedies" section for information on natural approaches.

NATURAL REMEDIES

Healthy lifestyle habits are important to prevent and
recover from prostate problems. The Five-A-Day Diet
(page 21) will provide you with essential nutrition.
Regular exercise and a thorough supplement program
are also important. If you have a prostate problem,
there are several natural products that enhance prostate health, as listed in the table below. Discuss them
with your health-care provider.

Natural Remedy	Dosage	Comments
Multivitamin/ mineral	See pages 14 to 20.	See pages 14 to 20.
Saw palmetto Propalmex; Proleve; Prostate SP; Prolynium	160 mg, 2 times daily; For the name brands given: 1 tablet, 2 times daily	Be sure that product is standardized to 85- to 95-percent fatty acids and sterol (also called liposterolic compounds). May take up to 60 days for full effectiveness to be experienced.

Propalmex and *Proleve* also contain zinc and pumpkin seed extract, which may be helpful. In addition, *Proleve* has a small amount of vitamin B$_6$. *Prostate SP* and *Prolynium* contain lycopene, an antioxidant from tomatoes that may have additional health benefits for the prostate.

Psoriasis

See also Skin Problems.

This common condition is characterized by dry, well-circumscribed, silvery, scaling patches of skin. Psoriasis most frequently affects the scalp, ears, back, arms, elbows, legs, and knees. It is chronic, coming and going over a lifetime, and varies in intensity. Specific factors can bring on an attack, some of which are: stress; nervous tension; severe sunburn; viral or bacterial infection; certain drugs, such as beta-blockers, chloroquine, and lithium; and irritation by external factors such as poison ivy.

Usually, the earlier in life this condition begins, the more severe it will be. In some people, psoriasis is less intense during the summer, as sunlight is helpful. There is no cure for psoriasis but, in most instances, the condition can be controlled.

OTC REMEDIES

The following table lists OTC products that are helpful

in reducing and/or relieving the symptoms of psoriasis. Always read the label before using a product.

OTC Remedy	Application	Comments
Caldecort Cream/Spray	As directed on label.	Also available in *Light Cream*. Reduces inflammation. Further skin irritation due to use of this product is uncommon. Do not use if you are allergic to any cortisone products.
Cortaid Cream/ Ointment/ Spray	As directed on label.	The regular- and maximum-strength formulas are available in cream and ointment forms, while the maximum-strength formula is also available in spray form. Reduces inflammation. Further skin irritation due to use of this product is uncommon. Do not use if you are allergic to any cortisone products.
Cortizone for Kids Anti-Itch Creme	As directed on label.	Reduces inflammation. Further skin irritation due to use of this product is uncommon. Do not use if you are allergic to any cortisone products.
Cortizone-5 Creme/Ointment	As directed on label.	Same comments as *Cortizone for Kids Anti-Itch Creme.*
Cortizone-10 Creme/Ointment	As directed on label.	Same comments as *Cortizone for Kids Anti-Itch Creme.*
Eucerin Creme	As directed on label.	Gently and effectively treats dryness.
Psoriasin Gel	As directed on label.	A coal-tar gel that may bring relief.

NATURAL REMEDIES

To obtain relief from psoriasis, it helps to avoid fats, sugar, processed foods, white flour, and citrus fruits. Eat a diet that contains 50-percent raw foods. Furthermore, add fish to your diet. For natural topical and supplement remedies, see the table below. An alternative/complementary medical practitioner may also help if your present course of action is not bringing results.

Natural Remedy	Application/ Dosage	Comments
Supplements		
Flaxseed oil	3 to 6 tbsp, daily	Contains essential fatty acids that promote healthy skin. Can also use a combination oil.
Vitamin E*	400 IU, daily	Take with a meal. Mixed tocopherols supplying 400 IU of d-alpha tocopherol are preferred. Can be used for long-term maintenance.
Topical Products		
Sarsparilla	Apply poultice to affected area, several times daily.	To make the poultice, heat fresh roots and wrap them in a sterile cloth.
Sea water	Apply to affected area with cotton, several times daily.	Has a soothing effect.

* It is important that the discussed nutrients be part of a basic vitamin/mineral regimen so that the total daily amount of each nutrient obtained from both a multivitamin/mineral and other supplements is approximately the dosage indicated above.

Rashes

See also Dermatitis; Jock Itch; Poison Ivy, Oak, Sumac; Psoriasis; Skin Problems.

A rash is an area of inflamed skin, whether in the form of spots or a solid redness. In general, rashes are temporary and may be either localized (affecting only a small area of skin) or generalized (covering the entire body). They can occur for a wide variety of reasons: as a symptom of a fever or another acute illness like chickenpox or scarlet fever; as an allergic reaction to a plant, food, drug, or environmental chemical; as part of a chronic skin disorder such as psoriasis or eczema; or even from an insect bite.

Itching is commonly associated with rashes. There are a number of over-the-counter products available that can treat this condition. It is rare that a rash is a symptom of a very serious health problem, yet it is important to identify the culprit so that you can best treat the primary problem. If you cannot trace the cause yourself, or if your rash results in significant pain, infection, or simply persists, see a dermatologist.

OTC REMEDIES

The following table lists products that are effective in combatting skin irritations. There are quite a few options for controlling itch and inflammation. If skin is broken, however, simply keeping the affected area clean and covered is likely to be the best solution.

These products are for external use only; avoid contact with the eyes and call your Poison Control Center if any ingestion of the products occurs. If no improvement results after seven days of use, consult a doctor. Always read the label before using a product.

OTC Remedies	Application	Comments
A & D Ointment	As directed on label.	Topical skin astringent, protectant, and antiseptic (kills bacteria). Further skin irritation due to use of this product is uncommon.
Anusol HC-1 Anti-Itch Hydrocortisone Ointment	As directed on label.	Reduces inflammation; soothes pain and itch. No common side effects. Adverse reactions, including such effects as dizziness, vision problems, further irritation of skin, and anxiety, are unusual. Do not use this product if you are allergic to cortisone or any topical pain-relieving products.
Benadryl Itch Relief Cream/Spray/Gel	As directed on label.	Available in children's and maximum strength formulas. Reduces inflammation. Further skin irritation due to use of this product is uncommon.
BiCozene Creme	As directed on label.	Topical anti-infective. Further skin irritation due to use of this product is uncommon.
Caladryl Cream/Lotion	As directed on label.	Also available in a cream for children.
Caldecort Anti-Itch Cream/Spray	As directed on label.	Also available in a *Light Cream*. Reduces inflammation. Further skin irritation due

		to use of this product is uncommon. Do not use if you are allergic to any cortisone products.
Caldesene Medicated Ointment/Powder	As directed on label.	Kills fungus cells. The powder absorbs excess moisture. Keep it away from the face to avoid inhalation. Further skin irritation due to use of this product is uncommon.
Clocream Skin Protectant Cream	As directed on label.	Soothes and protects the affected area. Further skin irritation due to use of this product is uncommon.
Cortaid Cream/Ointment/ Spray	As directed on label.	The regular- and maximum-strength formulas are available in cream and ointment forms, while the maximum-strength formula is also available in spray form. Reduces inflammation. Further skin irritation due to use of this product is uncommon. Do not use if you are allergic to cortisone products.
Cortizone for Kids Anti-Itch Creme	As directed on label.	Reduces inflammation. Further skin irritation due to use of this product is uncommon. Do not use if you are allergic to cortisone products.
Cortizone-5 Creme/Ointment	As directed on label.	Same comments as Cortizone for Kids Anti-Itch Creme.
Cortizone-10 Creme/Ointment	As directed on label.	Also available in anal-itch formula. Same comments as Cortizone for Kids Anti-Itch Creme.

Desitin *Cornstarch* *Baby Powder* *(with Zinc Oxide)*	As directed on label.	Absorbs excess moisture and promotes healing. Keep powder away from face to avoid inhalation.
Eucerin Creme	As directed on label.	Gently and effectively treats dryness.
Preparation-H *Hydrocortisone* *Anti-Itch Cream*	As directed on label.	Reduces pain, swelling, itching. No common side effects. Adverse reactions, including such effects as dizziness, vision problems, further irritation of skin, and anxiety, are possible but not usual. Do not use this product if you are allergic to cortisone or any topical pain-relievers.

NATURAL REMEDIES

To relieve the discomforts of a rash that comes from a skin reaction, apply very hot, water-soaked compresses to the affected area for short periods of time. If you are not satisfied with using just a plain water compress, try soaking the compress in diluted Burrow's solution (available in most drug stores). Cool-water colloidal oatmeal soaks are also soothing to irritated skin. Colloidal oatmeal is widely available in drug stores; the *Aveeno* brand is well-known.

If itching occurs, a paste made from water and any of the following may prove helpful: cornstarch; baking soda; oatmeal; or Epsom salts. To make this paste, mix 1 teaspoon of water with 3 teaspoons of the dry ingredient. Applying pure aloe vera juice/gel to the affected area to relieve itchiness or burning is another option. Other topical natural remedies include watermelon rind, tofu, and buttermilk mixed with sea salt (1 tablespoon of the salt to every pint of the buttermilk).

To promote healthy skin, drink lots of water and juices. In addition, consume a diet that is 50-percent raw foods. Follow a healthy diet, such as the Five-A-Day Diet (see page 21) or another diet recommended by a trained nutritionist. To help alleviate rashes that are associated with chronic skin disorders such as dermatitis or psoriasis, please see those individual sections. Good rest is also very important to skin health. For information on supplementation, see the table below.

Natural Remedy	Dosage	Comments
Flaxseed oil	Up to 1 tablespoon (or 1 to 3 teaspoons), daily	Helps to maintain proper fatty acid balance, promoting healthy skin.
Multivitamin/mineral,* including antioxidants	See pages 14 to 20.	See pages 14 to 20.
Vitamin A*	25,000 IU, daily	Take with a meal. Your *total* intake, including that amount provided by your multivitamin/mineral, should equal this dose. High doses of vitamin A should not be taken long term, as toxicity can result.
Vitamin E*	400 IU, daily	Take with a meal. Mixed tocopherols supplying 400 IU of d-alpha tocopherol are preferred. Can be used for long-term maintenance. General antioxidant for maintaining healthy skin.

Zinc*	30 mg, daily	Take with a meal. Doses in excess of 100 mg can depress immune function. If your multivitamin/mineral already contains this amount of zinc, there is no need for further supplementation.

* It is important that the discussed nutrients be part of a basic vitamin/mineral regimen so that the total daily amount of each nutrient obtained from both a multivitamin/mineral and other supplements is approximately the dosage indicated above.

Seborrhea

See Dermatitis; Skin Problems.

Sinusitis

See also Congestion, Nasal.

This inflammatory condition occurs in the paranasal sinuses—the cavities within the bones that surround the nose. The sinuses fill with mucus and fluid. Sinusitis is usually caused by a viral, bacterial, or fungal infection or by an allergic reaction. Actually, bacteria are responsible for over 50 percent of sinusitis cases. Hay fever and food allergies may also cause sinusitis.

Acute and chronic sinusitis share similar signs and symptoms. In both cases, the area over the infected sinus may be swollen or tender. There may also be pain in the jaw and behind or between the eyes, earache, headache, and/or toothache. Some people experience fever or malaise, as well.

In some cases, steam inhalation can promote

drainage from the sinuses and improve the condition. Observe the color of the drainage; greenish or yellowish mucus indicates an infection, while clear fluid indicates there is probably no infection. Antibiotics may be necessary for both acute and chronic sinusitis. It is important to treat this condition because it can lead to asthma, bronchitis, pneumonia, or other serious disorders.

OTC REMEDIES

The products listed in the following chart are analgesics—substances that relieve or reduce pain. These products also combat fever. If you have experienced side effects from any nonprescription pain relievers, do not take any of these remedies without consulting your doctor. Always read the label before using a product.

OTC Remedy	Dosage	Comments
For Pain, Fever, Muscular Aches		
Acetaminophen *Drixoral Cold & Flu Extended-Release Tablets; Excedrin Aspirin-Free; Panadol; Sinarest Tablets; Sine-Off Caplets; Sinutab Caplets/ Tablets; Theraflu Flu, Cold & Cough Medicine; Tylenol; Tylenol Cold Medicine*	325 mg regular strength; generally, 500 mg extra strength	Do not drink alcohol and use products containing acetaminophen. The combination can cause liver damage. Do not take with other analgesics. Many of these remedies come in various strengths and formulas. For example, *Tylenol, Sinarest, Sinutab,* and *Theraflu* are available in formulas that are extra or maximum strength. Some products have non-drowsiness formulas, including *Sinarest, Sinutab, Sine-Off,* and *Theraflu.*

Multi Symptom Formula Caplets/Tablets		Also look for nighttime formulas, such as *Theraflu Maximum-Strength Nighttime*.
Aspirin (acetylsalicylic acid) *Alka-Seltzer Plus Sinus Medicine; Ascriptin; Bayer; Bufferin; Ecotrin; Empirin; Excedrin Extra Strength*	325 mg regular strength; generally, 500 mg extra strength	If pregnant, consult your doctor before taking products containing aspirin. Do not take products containing aspirin during the last three months of pregnancy. Children and teens should not use products containing aspirin for colds, flus, or chickenpox. Do not take products containing aspirin if you have asthma, stomach problems, gastric ulcers, bleeding problems, or if you are allergic to aspirin.
Ibuprofen *Advil; Advil Cold & Sinus; Arthritis Foundation Ibuprofen; Motrin IB; Motrin IB & Sinus; Nuprin*	200 mg	If pregnant, consult your doctor before taking this remedy. Do not take products containing this ingredient during the last three months of pregnancy. Do not take this ingredient if you are allergic to aspirin. Do not take this ingredient with any other analgesics. Consult your doctor before taking this remedy with prescription drugs.
Ketoprofen *Orudis KT*	12.5 mg	Same comments as Ibuprofen.
Naproxen sodium *Aleve*	220 mg	If pregnant, consult your doctor before taking this remedy. Do not take products containing this ingredient during the last three months of pregnancy. Do not take this ingredient with any other analgesics. Consult your doctor before taking this remedy with prescription drugs.

For General Cold and Sinus Symptoms

Actifed	As directed on label.	May cause some drowsiness and/or dryness of the mucous membranes. Look for a non-drowsy formula or take necessary precautions. Maintain fluid intake.
Dimetapp Elixir/Liqui-gels/Tablets	As directed on label.	May cause some headache, drowsiness, dryness and stinging of the mucous membranes. Look for a non-drowsy formula or take necessary precautions. Maintain fluid intake.
Drixoral Cold & Allergy Sustained Action Tablets	As directed on label.	Same comments as *Actifed*.
Efidac 24	As directed on label.	Same comments as *Actifed*.
Sudafed Caplets/Tablets/Liquid	As directed on label.	Available in various strengths and formulas, among which is a children's liquid. See above comments for Acetaminophen, as some formulas contain that ingredient. Same comments as *Actifed*.
Tavist-1 Tablets	As directed on label.	Same comments as *Actifed*.
Tavist-D Tablets	As directed on label.	Same comments as *Actifed*.
Triaminic Cold Tablets	As directed on label.	Same comments as *Actifed*.
Triaminic-12 Tablets	As directed on label.	Same comments as *Actifed*.

For Nasal Congestion

4-Way Nasal Spray	As directed on label.	Available in *Fast Acting* and *Long Lasting* formulas. No common side effects. Nasal irritation or dryness occasionally occurs.

Afrin Nasal Spray	As directed on label.	No common side effects. Nasal irritation or dryness occasionally occurs.
Cheracol Nasal Spray Pump	As directed on label.	No common side effects. Nasal irritation or dryness occasionally occurs.
Neo-Synephrine Nasal Sprays/ Drops	As directed on label.	Available in various strengths, including pediatric, mild, regular, extra strength, and maximum strength 12-hour. No common side effects. Dryness and irritation of the nasal passages occasionally occur.
Pediacare Infant's Decongestant Drops	As directed on label.	No common side effects. Stomach discomforts, dizziness, and more severe reactions occur only infrequently.
Vicks Sinex Nasal Spray	As directed on label.	No common side effects. Nasal irritation or dryness occasionally occur.

Sinusitis can cause considerable pain and discomfort. If you require a pain reliever, know that when used responsibly, acetaminophen, aspirin, ibuprofen, ketoprofen, and naproxen sodium are safe and effective. Look for single-ingredient products. If you have questions or concerns regarding the safety and effectiveness of any product, consult your doctor or pharmacist.

NATURAL REMEDIES

To combat sinusitis, eat a diet that contains 75-percent raw foods and eliminate salt. Drink lots of fluids to help cleanse your body and to promote drainage. It is important to consume adequate amounts of vitamins

A and C. In treating sinus infections, and other viral infections as well, the following herbs have proven helpful: echinacea; goldenseal; licorice. See the table below for more detail.

Natural Remedy	Dosage	Comments
Echinacea	*Dried herb:* 300 mg, 3 times daily, for 14 days; *Fluid extract:* ½ tsp, 3 times daily, for 14 days	Appears to lose its immune-boosting properties after a couple of weeks. Therefore, it is most effective when used as a temporary treatment upon the first signs of symptoms.
Goldenseal	As directed on label.	Has anti-inflammatory, anti-bacterial, antibiotic qualities. Do not take if pregnant. Do not take daily for over 1 week. If allergic to ragweed, you may be sensitive to this herb. Use with caution.
Vitamin A*	10,000 to 25,000 IU, daily	Take with a meal. 10,000 IU is safe for long-term maintenance; higher doses should not be taken for longer than 14 days. Vitamin A deficiency can be the cause of sinusitis.
Vitamin C*	*First 10 days of infection:* 1,000 mg, 3 times daily; *For maintenance:* 500 mg, 2 times daily	Helps to fight infection. Safe for long-term maintenance.

* It is important that the discussed nutrients be part of a basic vitamin/mineral regimen so that the total daily amount of each nutrient obtained from both a multivitamin/mineral and other supplements is approximately the dosage indicated above.

Skin Problems

See also Acne; Dermatitis; Psoriasis; Rashes.

The skin—the body's largest organ—is the body's first line of defense against the microorganisms and other environmental substances and conditions that threaten the integrity of the body. The outer layer of the skin is called the epidermis; the middle layer, the dermis; and the inner layer, the subcutaneous layer. Allergies, foods, chemicals, drugs, plants, animals, sun, wind, and a thousand other factors can cause the skin to break out in rashes, acne, and other conditions that produce flaking, scaling, redness, and a host of different symptoms. Among the many common skin problems or dermatological conditions are dry skin, oily skin, rosacea, intertrigo, and sebaceous cysts.

Healthy skin requires a balance of water and oil in the cells. Dry skin occurs when cells are dehydrated and/or the production of sebum—skin oil—is inadequate. Poor nutrition, heredity, the sun, certain medications (such as diuretics), and exposure to harsh agents and elements can cause dry skin. Symptoms include a dull hue to the skin, discolorations or spotting, peeling, flaking, scaling, lines, tightness, and enlarged pores.

Oily skin involves an overproduction of sebum. The excess oil tends to clog pores, often resulting in blemishes. This condition can be due to heredity, diet, hormones, and/or hot and humid weather. The greasy look, enlarged pores, and common pimples that accompany oily skin are frustrating. But on the good

side, skin that produces considerable oil is not likely to
wrinkle or discolor prematurely.

Rosacea, or chronic reddening of the skin, frequently affects the nose, forehead, cheekbones, and
chin. If pustules appear at all, they will do so on the
nose. It is not known for certain what causes this condition, but stress, alcohol, sunlight, excessive heat or
cold, very hot liquids, and even spicy foods are suspected of being factors that worsen it. Tetracycline, an
antibiotic, may be needed to control this skin problem.

Intertrigo results from the friction of skin against
skin and is common on the inner thighs, underarms,
groin area, and breasts. Bacteria and yeast may also
cause this problem. The affected skin is likely to be
red, moist, and may give off an odor. There may also
be blisters or scales. Intertrigo can usually be resolved
by keeping the affected area clean and dry and by
minimizing skin friction. In some cases, weight reduction is the best way to solve this problem.

Sebaceous cysts are small nodules located just
beneath the skin surface. They are filled with sebum
and proteins from the skin. This condition frequently
occurs on the scalp, face, and back. The growths are
firm, but don't usually hurt unless an infection forms.
Chronic infection is possible. If a cyst becomes large or
infected, see a doctor. It may have to be removed or
drained to prevent the spread of infection.

OTC REMEDIES

The following table lists a number of OTC products
that will help restore health to your skin. Always read
the label before using a product.

OTC Remedy	Application	Comments
For Dry Skin		
Alpha Keri Moisture-Rich Body Oil	As directed on label.	Be careful not to slip in the shower or tub after using.
Curel Therapeutic Moisturizing Cream/Lotion	As directed on label.	
Dermasil Dry Skin Treatment Cream/Lotion	As directed on label.	Available in regular and concentrated formulas.
Eucerin Creme/Lotion	As directed on label.	Also available in *Eucerin Plus Moisturizing Alpha Hydroxy Creme/Lotion*.
Keri Lotion	As directed on label.	
Lubriderm Creme/Lotion	As directed on label.	Also available in *Alpha Hydroxy Formula Cream/Lotion*.
For Irritated Skin		
A & D Ointment	As directed on label.	Topical skin astringent, protectant, and antiseptic (kills bacteria). Further skin irritation due to use of this product is uncommon.
Anusol HC-1 Anti-Itch Hydrocortisone Ointment	As directed on label.	Reduces inflammation; soothes pain and itch. No common side effects. Some individuals have adverse reactions, including such effects as dizziness, vision problems, further irritation of skin, and anxiety, but this occurs only infrequently. Do not use this product if you are allergic to any cortisone or topical pain-relieving products.

Benadryl Itch Relief Cream/Spray/Gel	As directed on label.	Available in children's and maximum strength formulas. Reduces inflammation. Further skin irritation due to use of this product is uncommon.
BiCozene Creme	As directed on label.	Topical anti-infective. Further skin irritation due to use of this product is uncommon.
Caladryl Cream/Lotion	As directed on label.	Also available in a cream for children.
Caldecort Anti-Itch Cream/Spray	As directed on label.	Also available in a *Light Cream*. Reduces inflammation. Further skin irritation due to use of this product is uncommon. Do not use if you are allergic to any cortisone products.
Caldesene Medicated Ointment/Powder	As directed on label.	Kills fungus cells. The powder absorbs excess moisture. Keep it away from the face to avoid inhalation.
Clocream Skin Protectant Cream	As directed on label.	Soothes and protects the affected area. Further skin irritation due to use of this product is uncommon.
Cortaid Cream/Ointment/ Spray	As directed on label.	The regular- and maximum-strength formulas are available in cream and ointment forms, while the maximum-strength formula is also available in spray form. Reduces inflammation. Further skin irritation due to use of this product is uncommon. Do not use if you are allergic to cortisone products.

Cortizone for Kids Anti-Itch Creme	As directed on label.	Reduces inflammation. No common side effects. Further skin irritation due to use of this product is uncommon. Do not use if you are allergic to cortisone products.
Cortizone-5 Creme/Ointment	As directed on label.	Same comments as *Cortizone for Kids Anti-Itch Creme*.
Cortizone-10 Creme/Ointment/ Liquid	As directed on label.	Regular and anal-itch formulas are available in creme and ointment form. The scalp-itch formula is in liquid form. Same comments as *Cortizone for Kids Anti-Itch Creme*.
Desitin Cornstarch Baby Powder (with Zinc Oxide)	As directed on label.	Absorbs excess moisture and promotes healing. Keep powder away from face to avoid inhalation. Do not use on broken skin; see a doctor if there is no improvement after 7 days.
Preparation-H Hydrocortisone Anti-Itch Cream	As directed on label.	Reduces pain, swelling, itching. No common side effects. Adverse reactions, such as dizziness, vision problems, further irritation of skin, and anxiety, are possible but unusual. Do not use this product if you are allergic to any topical pain relievers.

NATURAL REMEDIES

A healthy diet usually translates into healthy skin; we recommend the Five-A-Day Diet (page 21). In order to prevent skin problems, drink plenty of water (8 ounces every hour, if you are trying to remedy skin problems) and juices, do not smoke, and take a good multivitamin/mineral that contains 25,000 IU of vitamin A. Avoid fried and junk foods, animal fat, excess sun exposure, soft drinks, sugar, and chocolate. Good rest is very important to skin health, as well.

If dry hands is your major problem, many people find that the cooking product *Crisco* is wonderful as a hand cream. For general skin health, there are a number of helpful nutrients and natural products, as detailed in the following table.

Natural Remedy	Application/ Dosage	Comments
For Dry Skin		
Aloe vera	Massage a small amount into dry area.	Has healing properties, as well as moisturizing benefits.
Vitamin E oil	Massage a small amount into dry area.	May be used as often as desired.
For General Skin Health		
Flaxseed oil	1 tbsp, daily	Source of omega-3 fatty acid, which may be beneficial to maintaining healthy skin. Many people find this remedy very effective.
Multivitamin/ mineral* with antioxidants	See pages 14 to 20.	See pages 14 to 20.
Vitamin A*	25,000 IU, daily	Take with a meal. Your *total* intake, including that amount provided by your multivitamin/mineral, should equal this dose. High doses of vitamin A should not be taken long term, as toxicity can result.
Vitamin E*	400 IU, daily	Take with a meal. Mixed tocopherols supplying 400 IU of d-alpha tocopherol

		are preferred. Can be used for long-term maintenance. General antioxidant for maintaining healthy skin.
Zinc*	Up to 30 mg, daily	Take with a meal. Doses in excess of 100 mg can depress immune function. Helps maintain healthy skin.

* It is important that the discussed nutrients be part of a basic vitamin/mineral regimen so that the total daily amount of each nutrient obtained from both a multivitamin/mineral and other supplements is approximately the dosage indicated above.

Sleep Disorders

See Chronic Fatigue Syndrome (CFS); Fatigue; Insomnia.

Sore Throat

The pain, burning, scratchiness, and aching of a sore throat can be caused by a wide variety of irritants that adversely affect the mucous membranes of the throat and mouth. Viruses and bacteria are common causes of sore throat. Often, a sore throat accompanies another condition, such as the flu, common cold, tonsillitis, or sinusitis. In addition, the following situations and irritants can make your throat sore: loud talking; a chronic cough; dust; smoke; fumes in the air; allergies; extremely hot food and drink; and infections of the teeth and gums. Hoarseness is a frequent symptom of sore throat.

Be sure to see a doctor if any of the following occur: your sore throat persists for more than two days; your sore throat is accompanied by a fever of 101°F; the glands in your neck are swollen; white patches appear on tonsils or in the tonsil area; a reddish rash appears on the trunk of the body; you have a history of rheumatic fever; or you have been exposed to either strep throat or mononucleosis. In addition, see a doctor if sore throats have been recurring and have not been previously treated by a physician.

OTC REMEDIES

In the following table, the products listed underneath and including acetaminophen, aspirin, ibuprofen, ketoprofen, and naproxen sodium are analgesics—substances that relieve or reduce pain. If you have experienced side effects from any nonprescription pain relievers, do not take any of these remedies without consulting your doctor. Always read the label before using a product.

OTC Remedy	Dosage	Comments
For Pain Relief		
Acetaminophen *Excedrin Aspirin-Free; Panadol; Tylenol*	325 mg regular strength; generally, 500 mg extra strength	Do not drink alcohol and use products containing acetaminophen. The combination can cause liver damage. Do not take with other analgesics. Some of these products, such as *Tylenol,* are available in regular, junior, and extra strength.

Aspirin (acetylsalicylic acid) *Ascriptin; Bayer; Bufferin; Ecotrin; Empirin; Excedrin Extra Strength*	325 mg regular strength; generally, 500 mg extra strength	If pregnant, consult your doctor before taking products containing aspirin. Do not take products containing aspirin during the last three months of pregnancy. Children and teens should not use products containing aspirin for colds, flus, or chickenpox. Do not take products containing aspirin if you have asthma, stomach problems, gastric ulcers, bleeding problems, or if you are allergic to aspirin.
Ibuprofen *Advil; Arthritis Foundation Ibuprofen; Motrin IB; Nuprin*	200 mg	If pregnant, consult your doctor before taking this remedy. Do not take products containing this ingredient during the last three months of pregnancy. Do not take this ingredient if you are allergic to aspirin. Do not take this ingredient with any other analgesics. Consult your doctor before taking this remedy with prescription drugs.
Ketoprofen *Orudis KT*	12.5 mg	Same comments as Ibuprofen.
Naproxen sodium *Aleve*	220 mg	If pregnant, consult your doctor before taking this remedy. Do not take products containing this ingredient during the last three months of pregnancy. Do not take this ingredient with any other analgesics. Consult your doctor before taking this remedy with prescription drugs.

For Cold Symptom Relief

Acetaminophen *Children's Tylenol Cold Multi-Symptom Chewable Tablets/Liquid; Comtrex Maximum-Strength Multi-Symptom Cold Reliever; Contac Severe Cold & Flu Non-Drowsy Caplets*	As directed on label.	Do not drink alcohol and use products containing acetaminophen. The combination can cause liver damage. Do not take with other analgesics.
Aspirin (acetylsalicylic acid) *Alka-Seltzer Cold Medicine*	As directed on label.	If pregnant, consult your doctor before taking products containing aspirin. Do not take products containing aspirin during the last three months of pregnancy. Children and teens should not use products containing aspirin for colds, flus, or chickenpox. Do not take products containing aspirin if you have asthma, stomach problems, gastric ulcers, bleeding problems, or if you are allergic to aspirin.

For Cough and Cold Symptom Relief

Acetaminophen *Children's Tylenol Cold Plus Cough Multi-Symptom Chewable Tablets/Liquid*	As directed on label.	Do not drink alcohol and use products containing acetaminophen. The combination can cause liver damage. Do not take with other analgesics.
Aspirin (acetylsalicylic acid) *Alka Seltzer Plus Cold & Cough*	As directed on label.	If pregnant, consult your doctor before taking products containing aspirin. Do not take products containing aspirin during the last three months of pregnancy.

		Children and teens should not use products containing aspirin for colds, flus, or chickenpox. Do not take products containing aspirin if you have asthma, stomach problems, gastric ulcers, bleeding problems, or if you are allergic to aspirin.
Halls Cough Suppressant Tablets	As directed on label.	Available in maximum-strength *(Halls Plus)*, as well as regular. Do not take for a persistent or chronic cough, or if you have excessive phlegm, unless otherwise directed by a doctor.
N'ICE Medicated Sugarless Sore Throat and Cough Lozenges	As directed on label.	Soothing lozenges that come in 6 varieties. Adults and children over 6 can take up to 10 lozenges a day. Same warnings as *Halls Cough Suppressant Tablets.*
For Sore Throat Relief Only		
Cheracol Sore Throat Spray	As directed on label.	Temporarily anesthetizes throat tissues.
Sucrets Lozenges	As directed on label.	Available in a variety of formulas, including: children's, regular, and maximum strength. Temporarily soothes throat tissues. Do not use with MAO inhibitors. Do not exceed maximum of 6 lozenges every 24 hours; for adults and children over 6. Same warnings as *Halls Cough Suppressant Tablets.*
Vicks Chloraseptic Sore Throat Lozenges/Spray	As directed on label.	Temporarily anesthetizes throat tissues.

Vicks *Cough Drops*	As directed on label.	Also available in extra strength. Same comments as *Halls Cough* *Suppressant Tablets.*

Sore throats can be very painful and you may decide that a pain reliever is necessary. If so, know that when used responsibly, acetaminophen, aspirin, ibuprofen, ketoprofen, and naproxen sodium are safe and effective. Look for single-ingredient products. If you have questions or concerns regarding the safety and effectiveness of any product, consult your doctor or pharmacist.

NATURAL REMEDIES

For occasional sore throat pain, gargle with warm salt water. Another option is to prepare a gargle mixture as follows: place 2 teaspoons of dried goldenseal and 2 teaspoons of sage leaves in a large mug. Pour boiling water over the mixture and then let it steep for ten minutes. Cool mixture to comfortable drinking temperature, then strain. Gargle as often as possible, or as desired. (See below for precautious concerning the use of goldenseal.)

Drink plenty of liquids, including fresh juices and raw honey with lemon. This will help to cleanse the body and restore health. See the table below for instructions on taking helpful herbs and other natural remedies. In addition, do not smoke. Smoking is both a cause and an aggravator of sore throat.

Natural Remedy	Dosage	Comments
Echinacea	*For standardized extract:* 300 mg, 3 times daily, for 10 days; *For brand name products:* as directed on label.	Standardized extract is available in capsules or tablets. Has anti-inflammatory and antiviral capacities. Appears to lose its effectiveness over time, so it should not be taken on a regular basis. Use as a short-term treatment. Do not use to treat immune deficiency diseases. Echinacea lozenges are also effective.
Goldenseal	As directed on label.	Has anti-inflammatory, anti-bacterial, antibiotic qualities. Do not take if pregnant. Do not take daily for over one week. If allergic to ragweed, you may be sensitive to this herb. Use with caution.
Vitamin C*	500 mg, 3 times daily, for 7 days, or maintain as daily regimen; if decreasing after 7 days, take 500 mg, 2 times daily, for 4 days, then maintain at 500 mg daily	These dosage instructions are for individuals who are routinely taking less than 500 mg of vitamin C, daily. Remember to consider the amount that you are receiving through your multivitamin/ mineral supplement.
Zinc Lozenges	*First day:* dissolve 1 lozenge under tongue every 2 hours; *Second day:* dissolve 1 lozenge under tongue every 4 hours; *Third through sixth days:* dissolve 1	Works best if taken at the first sign of sore throat. Some individuals experience mouth irritation from frequent use of zinc lozenges. Try different brands until you find the one that best suits you.

lozenge under tongue
every 6 hours

---

*It is important that the above-listed nutrients be part of a basic vitamin/mineral regimen so that the total daily amount of each nutrient obtained from both a multivitamin/mineral and other supplements is approximately the dosage indicated above.

Stretch Marks

See also Pregnancy-Related Problems.

Stretch marks are caused by rapid, excessive weight gain. Frequently, this occurs during pregnancy. When the skin is over-stretched, fibers in deep skin layers tear. As a result, wavy, reddish "stripes" may appear on the thighs, buttocks, breasts, and abdomen. Over time, the stripes turn white. Stretch marks never go away, but they do become less noticeable.

OTC REMEDIES

There are no OTC products that can fade stretch marks. However, a combination of natural substances may help to prevent them. See "Natural Remedies," below.

NATURAL REMEDIES

A mixture of virgin olive oil, aloe vera gel, vitamin E oil, and vitamin A oil applied to areas where stretch marks commonly appear can be very helpful in preventing this condition. The oily lotion will keep the skin lubricated, so that it does not pull and mark as easily if the body suddenly takes on extra weight.

Sunburn

Excessive exposure to ultraviolet rays burns the skin. These rays can harm the skin on hazy days, as well as on days without a cloud in the sky. The intensity of ultraviolet radiation varies with geographical location, season, time of day, weather, and individual susceptibility. Evidence indicates that damage to the earth's protective ozone layer, which protects living things from the ultraviolet rays, has increased the risks associated with sunburn and overexposure to sunlight.

Between the hours of 11 A.M. and 2 P.M., ultraviolet radiation is at its strongest. It is best to avoid being in the sun during those hours. A person's exposure to ultraviolet rays can double when out in the snow, on the water, or at the beach, so extra care is required. "Tanning" indicates that the skin has been damaged. Reddening is a sign of first-degree burns; reddening with water blisters indicates second-degree burns; burns with skin eruptions and fluid discharge signify third-degree burns and require immediate attention by a doctor in order to prevent serious skin damage and infection. In fact, see a doctor if sunburn is accompanied by nausea, chills, or fever, or if you feel faint, have blistered skin, or have intense itching.

OTC REMEDIES

The products listed in the first section of the following table are analgesics—substances that relieve or reduce pain. If you have experienced side effects from any nonprescription pain relievers, do not take any of these remedies without consulting your doctor. Always read the label before using a product. While there are topical products that are helpful for minor and moderate burns, severe burns require a doctor's attention.

OTC Remedy	Dosage	Comments
Oral Pain-Relieving Medications		
Acetaminophen *Excedrin Aspirin-Free; Panadol; Tylenol*	325 mg regular strength; generally, 500 mg extra strength	Do not drink alcohol and use products containing acetaminophen. The combination can cause liver damage. Do not take with other analgesics. Some of these products, such as *Tylenol,* are available in regular, junior, and extra strength.
Aspirin (acetylsalicylic acid) *Ascriptin; Bayer; Bufferin; Ecotrin; Empirin; Excedrin Extra Strength*	325 mg regular strength; generally, 500 mg extra strength	If pregnant, consult your doctor before taking products containing aspirin. Do not take products containing aspirin during the last three months of pregnancy. Children and teens should not use products containing aspirin for colds, flus, or chickenpox. Do not take products containing aspirin if you have asthma, stomach problems, gastric ulcers, bleeding problems, or if you are allergic to aspirin.
Ibuprofen *Advil; Arthritis Foundation Ibuprofen; Motrin IB; Nuprin*	200 mg	If pregnant, consult your doctor before taking this remedy. Do not take products containing this ingredient during the last three months of pregnancy. Do not take this ingredient if you are allergic to aspirin. Do not take this ingredient with any other analgesics.

		Consult your doctor before taking this remedy with prescription drugs.
Ketoprofen *Orudis KT*	12.5 mg	Same comments as Ibuprofen.
Naproxen sodium *Aleve*	220 mg	If pregnant, consult your doctor before taking this remedy. Do not take products containing this ingredient during the last three months of pregnancy. Do not take this ingredient with any other analgesics. Consult your doctor before taking this remedy with prescription drugs.

Topical Products

Americaine Topical Anesthetic Spray/First Aid Ointment	As directed on label.	Temporarily blocks the pain messages sent from the skin to the brain. Further skin irritation (possibly including hives) due to use of this product is uncommon.
BiCozene Creme	As directed on label.	Topical anti-infective. Further skin irritation due to use of this product is uncommon.
Clocream Skin Protectant Cream	As directed on label.	Soothes and protects the affected area. Further skin irritation due to use of this product is uncommon.
Eucerin Creme	As directed on label.	Gently and effectively moisturizes skin. Further skin irritation due to use of this product is uncommon.

Sunburn can cause considerable pain and you may feel that a pain reliever is necessary. If so, know that when used responsibly, acetaminophen, aspirin, ibuprofen, ketoprofen, and naproxen sodium are safe and effective. Look for single-ingredient products. If you have questions or concerns regarding the safety and effectiveness of any product, consult your doctor or pharmacist. Certain product ingredients can put your skin at greater risk. It is important to note that some health professionals hold the following opinion:

- Products containing any of the following may make your skin more sensitive to the sun and worsen sunburn: naproxen sodium; diphenhydramine; phenylbutazone; ketoprofen; clemastine.

NATURAL REMEDIES

The most effective natural remedy for sunburn is to apply aloe vera gel (see table below) to the injured skin. In addition, a baking soda bath may be helpful; add 1 cup of baking soda to a lukewarm bath and soak for thirty minutes. Furthermore, the following table lists several natural remedies that will bring comfort and healing to your sunburn.

Natural Remedy	Dosage/Application	Comments
Nutritional Supplements		
Multivitamin/mineral*	See pages 14 to 20.	See pages 14 to 20. If you do not usually supplement with vitamins and minerals daily, this is a good time to start. Balancing your nutrition will help you heal more quickly and maintain better general health.

Vitamin C*	500 to 1,000 mg, 3 times daily, orally	Speeds healing. Safe for long-term maintenance.
Vitamin E*	400 IU, daily, orally	Take with a meal. Assists in skin health. Mixed tocopherols supplying 400 IU of d-alpha tocopherol are preferred. Can be used for long-term maintenance.
Topical Treatments		
Aloe vera gel	Apply to affected area as often as possible.	Provides soothing comfort. Be sure that the product contains 100-percent aloe vera.

* It is important that the discussed nutrients be part of a basic vitamin/mineral regimen so that the total daily amount of each nutrient obtained from both a multivitamin/mineral and other supplements is approximately the dosage indicated above.

Teething

See also Dental Problems.

Teething is the process that every infant experiences as his or her teeth grow and break through the gums. It usually occurs between the ages of six months and three years, but some children begin teething earlier, while others take a longer time. The extent of the discomfort involved is very dependent on the individual child. Some experience only mild pain that does not significantly affect their behavior or sleep patterns. However, other children go through considerable discomfort and are continually cranky, fatigued, and crying. Common symptoms are red and swollen gums, drooling, and the desire to put objects (including hands) in the mouth. If the child is experiencing fever and digestive problems, it is important to see a physician for guidance.

NATURAL REMEDIES

Be extra cautious with the use of OTCs when it comes to treating infants. Luckily, there are products that are specifically formulated for infant use, especially for teething woes. Always read the label before using a product.

OTC Remedy	Application	Comments
Baby Orajel Teething Pain Medicine	As directed on label.	Temporarily anesthetizes the affected area.
Baby Orajel Tooth & Gum Cleanser	As directed on label.	Keeps open gums and new teeth protected from bacterial attacks.

NATURAL REMEDIES

A baby is likely to find some relief by biting on cold, firm objects. Teething rings that can be kept refrigerated or frozen are helpful. So are hard foods like teething biscuits, bread crusts, and juice pops. Rubbing the gums with your finger and/or applying pure aloe vera gel may provide topical comfort. Also, keeping the child occupied with activities will help to distract him or her from the discomfort.

Tick Bites

See Insect Bites.

Tooth Decay

See Dental Problems.

Tooth-Grinding

See Bruxism.

Toothache

See also Dental Problems.

This condition is characterized by pain localized in a particular tooth. If the pain is provoked by sweets or cold, there is likely to be decay and/or a cavity (*caries*) that has not yet involved a nerve. This type of pain is usually transitory. Pain that is brought on by heat generally indicates caries that has reached the nerve. This pain usually lasts for a longer time.

It is best to avoid foods and liquids that bring on pain, to use a mild painkiller, and to seek treatment from a dentist. By treating this condition as soon as possible, future problems can be prevented. Advanced decay can lead to the development of an abcess underneath a tooth, which can be very painful (although sometimes abcesses go completely undetected until x-rays are taken) and even dangerous. If an abcess ruptures, serious infection can spread.

OTC REMEDIES

The following table lists OTC products that work

well when it comes to alleviating toothache pain. The products in the first section are analgesics—substances that relieve or reduce pain. These products also combat fever, which often accompanies an infection. If you have experienced side effects from any nonprescription pain relievers, do not take any of these remedies without consulting your doctor. The item listed under "Topical Product" can be applied directly to the painful area, in order to provide immediate soothing. Always read the label before using a product.

OTC Remedy	Dosage/Application	Comments
Oral Pain-Relieving Medications		
Acetaminophen *Excedrin Aspirin-Free; Panadol; Tylenol*	325 mg regular strength, generally, 500 mg extra strength	Do not drink alcohol and use products containing acetaminophen. The combination can cause liver damage. Do not take with other analgesics. Some products, such as *Tylenol*, are available in regular, junior, and extra strength.
Aspirin (acetylsalicylic acid) *Ascriptin; Bayer; Bufferin; Ecotrin; Empirin; Excedrin Extra Strength*	325 mg regular strength; generally, 500 mg extra strength	If pregnant, consult your doctor before taking products containing aspirin. Do not take products containing aspirin during the last three months of pregnancy. Children and teens should not use products containing aspirin for colds, flus, or chickenpox. Do not take products containing aspirin if you have asthma, stomach problems, gastric ulcers, bleeding problems, or if you are allergic to aspirin.

Ibuprofen *Advil; Arthritis* *Foundation* *Ibuprofen;* *Motrin IB;* *Nuprin*	200 mg	If pregnant, consult your doctor before taking this remedy. Do not take products containing this ingredient during the last three months of pregnancy. Do not take this ingredient if you are allergic to aspirin. Do not take this ingredient with any other analgesics. Consult your doctor before taking this remedy with prescription drugs.
Ketoprofen *Orudis KT*	12.5 mg	Same comments as Ibuprofen.
Naproxen **sodium** *Aleve*	220 mg	If pregnant, consult your doctor before taking this remedy. Do not take products containing this ingredient during the last three months of pregnancy. Do not take this ingredient with any other analgesics. Consult your doctor before taking this remedy with prescription drugs.
Topical Product		
Benzocaine *Orajel Maximum-* *Strength* *Toothache* *Medicine*	Applied directly to sore area, as directed on label.	Temporarily anesthetizes the sore area.

Toothache can cause considerable pain, and you may find it necessary to take a pain reliever. If so, know that when used responsibly, acetaminophen, aspirin, ibuprofen, ketoprofen, and naproxen sodium are safe and effective. Look for single-ingredient products. If you have questions or concerns regarding the

safety and effectiveness of any product, consult your
doctor or pharmacist.

NATURAL REMEDIES

If a toothache results from decay and cavities, there
are no natural substances that can cure the problem.
Again, see your dentist and remedy the cause of the
ache as soon as possible. However, good nutrition is a
must for healthy teeth and gums, and there are natural
substances that can help you to efficiently fight infection. In addition, some herbs and oils can soothe the
pain. See the table below for information. Also, rinsing
your mouth with warm saltwater ($^{1}/_{2}$ teaspoon of salt
per 8-ounce glass of water) can bring comfort to the
sore area.

Natural Remedy	Dosage/Application	Comments
Nutritional Supplements		
Multivitamin/mineral*	See pages 14 to 20.	See pages 14 to 20.
Vitamin A*	10,000 IU daily	Take with a meal. Necessary for maintaining healthy tissues.
Vitamin C*	500 mg, 3 times daily	Helps fight infection and promotes healing. Safe for long-term use.
Herbal Treatments		
Echinacea	1 to 2 tsp of tincture, in water.	Soothes discomfort; has anti-inflammatory and antiviral capacities. Take hourly until the pain subsides, or for 2 days. If pain persists, see your dentist.

| Goldenseal | ½ tsp, in water, 3 times daily. | Fights bacteria and decreases inflammation.
Do not take if pregnant.
Daily internal use should be limited to one week.
You may be sensitive to this herb if you are allergic to ragweed; use with caution. |

---

* It is important that the discussed nutrients be part of a basic vitamin/mineral regimen so that the total daily amount of each nutrient obtained from both a multivitamin/mineral and other supplements is approximately the dosage indicated above.

Urinary Tract Infection

See Cystitis; Vaginitis.

Vaginitis

See also Candidiasis; Yeast Infection.

This condition involves an inflammation of the vaginal lining. It can be caused by bacteria, yeast, or protozoa. In fact, about one-third of all vaginitis cases are caused by the protozoan *Trichomonas vaginalis*. Human papilloma virus (HMV) is also associated with some cases. Burning, itching, inflammation of the vaginal mucosa and the vulva, and fluid discharge are common symptoms of vaginitis. A certain amount of discharge is normal for a lot of women, but if you find that it occurs in large amounts, has a bad odor, or accompanies itching, burning, or pain, suspect vaginitis and see your doctor.

Frequent douching with chemical products may

contribute to vaginitis by altering the vagina's natural state. Tight, nonporous, nonabsorbent underwear can foster the growth of bacteria related to vaginitis. Poor personal hygiene heightens the risk of bacterial and fungal infection. Furthermore, some women are sensitive to spermicides, latex in condoms, or the substances used for diaphragms and coital lubricants. Vaginitis can be brought on by the use of oral contraceptives or antibiotics, both of which can destroy bacteria that the body needs to maintain health. Consult a doctor for help with this problem, and be sure to discuss any medications and contraceptives that you use.

OTC REMEDIES

You should treat vaginitis under your doctor's supervision. But to aid in cleansing the vagina, *Massingill Medicated Disposable Douche* is recommended. This is a water-and-vinegar douche, not a chemical solution.

NATURAL REMEDIES

An experienced nutritionist may suggest dietary changes that can help to eliminate this condition. In any case, the Five-A-Day Diet is a healthy program to follow (see page 21), as it will improve overall, long-term immune function. A diet free of sugar and yeast, and low in carbohydrates, will work to restore proper balance to the vagina. Keep the vaginal area clean and dry. Wear white cotton underwear that allows healthy air circulation. Applying vitamin E cream or oil to the inflamed area will help to relieve itching.

Varicose Veins

See also Hemorrhoids.

When the valves in the veins are not working properly, blood accumulates and stretches the veins. The resulting swollen, abnormally enlarged vessels are termed varicose veins, and are most often found in the legs. These prominent veins are usually bluish in color. Dull aches and pains that cause nagging discomfort commonly accompany this condition.

Varicose veins are common among: those who sit for prolonged periods, especially with legs crossed; those who do not exercise regularly; those who are overweight or pregnant; and those whose work entails heavy lifting. If you have swelling, leg sores, leg cramps, and/or a feeling of heaviness in the legs, consult a doctor. Furthermore, varicose veins can be an indication of underlying health problems (for example, constipation, heart problems), so medical attention is required. "Spider veins," which are thin, red capillaries that can be seen through the skin, are not cause for concern.

OTC REMEDY

There are no OTC products that can help treat or prevent varicose veins. However, see the following "Natural Remedies" section for some helpful natural approaches to this condition.

NATURAL REMEDIES

Exercise is very important for the prevention and

treatment of varicose veins; walking, swimming, and cycling are good ways to improve your circulation. Proper posture when sitting and standing also helps to maintain healthy blood flow. Avoid crossing your legs when sitting, and try not to sit or stand for long periods of time. Changing position and moving around keeps the blood moving.

It is beneficial to elevate your feet and legs above your heart for ten to fifteen minutes at night. Lie on your back on the floor and rest your legs on a chair or your bed. Another approach is to sleep with your feet slightly elevated by putting a pillow wedge under your feet or by raising the bottom end of your mattress several inches.

Constipation can be a cause of varicose veins, so be sure to consume a good amount of fiber. In general, a healthy diet will allow for healthier vascular conditions. Aim for a diet low in fat and refined carbohydrates, and high in fish, fresh fruits, and vegetables. The following table lists several natural supplements that will also help to prevent or treat varicose veins.

Natural Remedy	Dosage	Comments
Coenzyme Q_{10} (also called CoQ_{10} and ubiquinone)	100 mg, daily	Improves overall circulation, although it targets heart health more than other areas.
Grape-seed extract or Pine bark extract *Pycnogenol*	50 mg, daily	Helps to prevent, but not to treat, varicose veins. Grape-seed extract and pine bark extract are comparable substances.

Horse chestnut extract *Venostat*	50 mg, 2 times daily	Make sure that product is standardized to 16- to 21-percent Escin (sometimes spelled Aescin) content. Studies in Europe demonstrate the value of horse chestnut extract for strengthening the veins, decreasing leg and foot swelling, and helping to eliminate spider veins and some varicose veins. It is great for improving circulation.
Vitamin C*	500 to 1,000 mg, 3 times daily	Helps to strengthen blood vessels to prevent, but not treat, varicose veins. Safe for long-term maintenance.
Vitamin E*	400 IU, daily	Take with a meal. Improves circulation and tissue elasticity. Helps prevent blood clots from forming. Mixed tocopherols supplying 400 IU of d-alpha tocopherol are preferred. Can be used for long-term maintenance.

* It is important that the discussed nutrients be part of a basic vitamin/mineral regimen so that the total daily amount of each nutrient obtained from both a multivitamin/mineral and other supplements is approximately the dosage indicated above.

Vision Problems

See Eye problems.

Warts

Common warts are rough, irregular growths of skin that usually occur on the feet, hands, forearms, and face. They can be as small as a pinhead or as large as a bean. Warts can be raised or flat, wet or dry, skin color or darker than the person's skin. They are caused by viruses and are highly contagious. In fact, warts can be spread simply by picking at them or touching them. Sometimes they can be spread by shaving. Common warts are usually painless and will disappear on their own.

Plantar warts most often affect only the bottom of the feet and toes. These small and bumpy growths can look much like calluses, but they are often sensitive and can bleed if irritated. This type of wart generally does not spread to other locations.

Venereal warts, also called genital warts, are another story. Early detection of this condition is critical because the carrier may not know he or she has them and can spread them to others. These rough, bumpy growths may appear singly or in clusters around the groin, vagina, anus, penis, or scrotal area. They are sexually transmitted and highly contagious. If there is a suspicion of venereal warts, see a doctor. Women should see a gynecologist. Genital warts are associated with an increased cancer risk in women. If this condition is present, women may have to have repeated Pap smears for a period of time.

Do not self-diagnose and self-medicate warts. Have a doctor make a diagnosis as to what type of wart you have. If it is confirmed that you have common or plantar warts, there are several self-treatment options.

OTC REMEDIES

The following table lists OTC products that treat common and plantar warts. Always read the label before using any product.

OTC Remedy	Application	Comments
Compound W Gel/Liquid	As directed on label.	Works to break down and remove the outermost layer of skin, called the keratin. Do not use on open or infected skin. Common side effects include any of the following in the treated area: darkening of skin; heat; peeling; stinging. Occasionally, individuals experience more severe reactions, such as blistering, inflammation, or intense irritation. If this occurs, stop using the product and call your doctor. Do not use this product if you are allergic to salicylic acid or resorcinol. Consult a doctor before using this product if you have eczema, diabetes, or a disorder of the blood vessels. Consult a doctor before using this product if you are taking or using another medication.
Dr. Scholl's Wart Remover	As directed on label.	Same comments as *Compound W Gel/Liquid.*

| Duoplant Gel Wart Remover | As directed on label. | Same comments as *Compound W Gel/Liquid*. |
| Wart-Off Liquid | As directed on label. | Same comments as *Compound W Gel/Liquid*. |

NATURAL REMEDIES

A healthy diet is essential to restoring the proper immune function that will, in turn, help eradicate warts. We recommend the Five-A-Day Diet (see page 21). Also, as part of your dietary regimen, increase sulfur-containing amino acids in the diet, which can be obtained through such foods as asparagus, citrus fruits, eggs, garlic, and onions. Desiccated liver tablets are another good source. And plenty of vitamin C will help to boost your immune system and therefore fight the viruses causing the warts.

Some people find that simply bathing the wart in hot water—120°F to 130°F—resolves the problem. See the following table for more information on natural remedies.

Natural Remedy	Dosage/Application	Comments
Nutritional Supplements		
Multivitamin/ mineral	See pages 14 to 20.	See pages 14 to 20. Nutrient balance is very important for healthy skin and proper immune function.
Topical Treatments		
Castor oil and baking soda	A paste, applied to the wart.	Might remove the wart within several weeks.
Garlic	1 crushed clove, applied to the wart.	A traditional remedy that may work within 1 to 2 weeks.

Yeast Infections

See also Candidiasis; Vaginitis.

When a fungus (for example, *Candida albicans*) grows in the body, yeast infections occur and can cause vaginitis. Vaginal burning, itching, and discharge are common symptoms of a yeast infection. This condition will affect almost every woman at some time in her life. And yeast infections often recur if immunity is not boosted.

Women with diabetes are more prone to yeast infections. The use of oral contraceptives and some antibiotics may also make a woman more susceptible to this condition because these products disrupt the natural environment of the vagina. Yeast infections are quite common during pregnancy, as well. And women who have infants or who care for infants should be aware that it is easy to transmit *Candida albicans* to these children. Consult a doctor for a diagnosis.

Commercial douches and sprays are generally unhealthy for the pH balance of the vaginal environment and can do more harm than good. So it is best to get a health-care professional's guidance concerning a treatment process.

OTC REMEDIES

The following table lists OTC products that are helpful in the treatment of vaginal yeast infections. Keep in mind that OTC products are not necessarily the best step in treating this condition, as they can further disrupt the vagina's pH balance. Always read the label before using any product.

OTC Remedy	Application	Comments
Clotrimazole *Gyne-Lotrimin Vaginal Cream/ Vaginal Inserts/ Combination Pack; Mycelex-7 Vaginal Cream/ Vaginal Inserts/ Combination Pack*	As directed on label.	Kills fungus cells. No common side effects. Further vaginal irritation, swelling, and discharge are unusual.
Miconazole nitrate *Monistat 7 Vaginal Cream/ Vaginal Inserts*	As directed on label.	Same comments as Clotrimazole.

NATURAL REMEDIES

To prevent or treat vaginal yeast infections, consume a diet low in sugar, carbohydrates, and yeast. Eat live-culture yogurt, which will restore some healthy bacteria to the body. The following table includes several suggestions involving natural nutrients and substances that may be of further help.

Natural Remedy	Dosage	Comments
Acidophilus	As directed on label.	Helps restore healthy bacteria to the vagina. Purchase products that have been refrigerated, to ensure potency.
Multivitamin/ mineral	See pages 14 to 20.	See pages 14 to 20. Vitamin and mineral balance is essential to vaginal health.

Appendix A: Resources

Below are listed organizations and services that can provide you with further information concerning many of the conditions and treatments discussed in this book. Phone numbers, addresses, and websites are subject to change.

GENERAL HEALTH INFORMATION:

American Medical Association (AMA)
515 North State Street
Chicago, IL 60610
312–464–5000

National Health Information Center
PO Box 1133
Washington, DC 20013-1133
800–336–4797; 301–565–4167
Website: http://www.nhic-nt.health.org
E-mail: nhicinfo@health.org

ORGANIZATIONS FOR SPECIFIC CONDITIONS:

American Academy of Allergy, Asthma, and Immunology
611 East Wells Street
Milwaukee, WI 53202
800–822–ASMA

American Anorexia/Bulimia Association
  Hot Line
212–501–8351

American Council for Headache
  Education (ACHE)
875 Kings Highway, Suite 200
Woodbury, NJ 08096
800–255–ACHE
Website: www.achenet.org

American Dental Association
211 East Chicago Avenue
Chicago, IL 60611
312–440–2500

American Heart Association
7272 Greenville Avenue
Dallas, TX 75231
1–800–AHA–USA1

American Menopause Foundation, Inc.
The Empire State Building
350 Fifth Avenue, Suite 2822
New York, NY 10118
212–714–2398

American Sleep Disorders
6301 Bandel Rd., Suite 101
Rochester, MN 55901
507–287–6006

Anorexia Nervosa and Associated Disorders (ANAD)
PO Box 7
Highland Park, IL 60035
847–831–3438
Anxiety Disorders Association of America
11900 Parklawn Drive, Suite 100
Rockville, MD 20852-2624
301–231–9350

Arthritis Foundation
1314 Spring Street NW
Atlanta, GA 30309
800–283–7800

Asthma and Allergy Foundation of America
1125 15th Street NW, Suite 305
Washington, DC 20005
800–7–ASTHMA; 202–466–7643
(Monday to Friday, 9AM to 5PM EST)
Website: www.aafa.org

Chronic Fatigue and Immune Dysfunction Syndrome
(CFIDS) Foundation
PO Box 220398
Charlotte, NC 28222-0398
800–442–3437

Food Allergy Network
10400 Eaton Place, Suite 107
Fairfax, VA 22030-5647
703–691–3179

Herpes Resource Center
PO Box 13827
Research Triangle Park, NC 27709
919–361–8488
800–230–6039 for a representative who can give information on written material.
800–653–4325 for recorded messages about herpes and other sexually transmitted diseases.

National Alopecia Areata Foundation
710 C Street, Suite 11
San Rafael, CA 94901
415–456–4644

National Asthma Center Lung Line
1400 Jackson Street
Denver, CO 80206
800–222–LUNG

National Chronic Pain Outreach Association
7979 Old Georgetown Road, Suite 100
Bethesda, MD 20814
301–652–4948

National Digestive Diseases Information Clearinghouse
2 Information Way
Bethesda, MD 20892–3570
301–654–3810

National Eating Disorders Organization
6655 South Yale
Tulsa, OK 74136
918–481–4044

National Eye Institute (NEI)
National Institutes of Health
Building 31, Room 6A32
31 Center Drive, MSC 2510
Bethesda, MD 20892–2510
301–496–5248

National Foundation for Depressive Illness
PO Box 2257
New York, NY 10116
800–248–4344

National Headache Foundation
428 West Saint James Place, 2nd Floor
Chicago, IL 60614
800–843–2256

National Institute of Allergies and Infectious Diseases
National Institutes of Health
Building 31, Room 7A50
31 Center Drive, MSC 2520
Bethesda, MD 20892–2520
301–496–5717

National Mental Health Association
1021 Prince Street
Alexandria, VA 22314
800–969–6642
PMS Access
PO Box 9362
Madison, WI 53715
800–222–4767; 608–833–4767

NUTRITION AND ALTERNATIVE/ COMPLEMENTARY MEDICINE ASSOCIATIONS:

American Dietetic Association
216 West Jackson Boulevard, Suite 800
Chicago, IL 60606–6995
800–366–1655

American Association of Nutritional Consultants
810 South Buffalo Street
Warsaw, IN 46580
888–828–2262

American Botanical Council
PO Box 144345
Austin, TX 78714-4345
512–331–8868
Website: http://www.herbalgram.org

American Chiropractic Association
1701 Clarendon Boulevard
Arlington, VA 22209
800–986–4636

American Holistic Medical Association
6728 Old McLean Village Drive
McLean, VA 22101
703–556–9245
(send $5.00 for a national referral directory of practitioners of herbal medicine)

American Massage Therapy Association
820 Davis Street, Suite 100
Evanston, IL 60201-4444
847–864–0123

Center for Nutrition and Dietetics Consumer Hot Line
800–366–1655

Herb Research Foundation
1007 Pearl Street, Suite 200
Boulder, CO 80302–9953
800–748–2617; 303–449–2265
Fax: 303–449–7849
Website: http://www.herbs.org

International Association of Yoga Therapists
20 Sunnyside Avenue, Suite A243
Mill Valley, CA 94941
415–332–2478

International and American Associations of Clinical Nutritionists (IAACN)
5200 Keller Springs Road, Suite 410
Dallas, TX 75248
972–250–2829
Fax: 972–250–0233

International Chiropractors Association
1110 North Glebe Road, Suite 1000
Arlington, VA 22201
703–528–5000

National Acupuncture and Oriental Medicine Alliance
14637 Starr Road, SE
Olalla, WA 98359
253–851–6896

National Institutes of Health
Office of Alternative Medicine
9000 Rockville Pike
Building 31, Room 5B-38
Bethesda, MD 20892
301–402–2466
Fax: 301–402–4741
Website: www.dietarysupplements.info.nih.gov

Price-Pottenger Nutrition Foundation
PO Box 2614
La Mesa, CA 91943
619–582–4168
(membership fees start at $25)

Transcendental Meditation
888–532–7686
(An operator in your state will answer and provide
you with information on instructors in your location.)

ADDITIONAL HELPFUL WEBSITES:

http://www.dole5aday.com
http://www.healthy.net
http://www.herbalgram.org.directory.html
http://www.herbweb.com.encyclopedia
http://www.herblore.com
http://www.nextpharmaceuticals.com
http://www.realtime.net/anr

Appendix B:
Personal Medical Form

_____   _____
Name   Date of Birth

DAILY MEDICATIONS

_____   _____
_____   _____
_____   _____

DAILY SUPPLEMENTS
Vitamins/Minerals: **Herbs and Other:**

_____   _____
_____   _____
_____   _____

ALLERGIES AND SENSITIVITIES
Medications: **Environmental Factors:**

_____   _____
_____   _____
_____   _____

Foods and Beverages: **Other:**

_____   _____
_____   _____
_____   _____

SPECIAL NUTRITIONAL NEEDS

(examples—supplemental iron for iron-deficiency anemia; low-sugar diet for diabetes)

_____   _____
_____   _____
_____   _____
_____   _____

VACCINATIONS/BOOSTERS

Vaccine: **Date:**   **Age:**

_____   _____   _____
_____   _____   _____
_____   _____   _____
_____   _____   _____
_____   _____   _____
_____   _____   _____
_____   _____   _____
_____   _____   _____

SIGNIFICANT LIFESTYLE HABITS

(examples—smoking; drinking alcohol; dependency on caffeine)

Habit: **Date Began:**   **Frequency/ Amount:**

_____   _____   _____
_____   _____   _____
_____   _____   _____
_____   _____   _____

SIGNIFICANT ILLNESSES/SURGERIES

Condition: **Date:** **Treatment:**

_____ _____ _____

_____

_____ _____ _____

_____

_____ _____ _____

_____

_____ _____ _____

_____

_____ _____ _____

_____

_____ _____ _____

TRAUMATIC EMOTIONAL EVENTS

(examples—death of loved one; divorce; depression; anxiety)

Event: **Date:** **Medical Treatment, if any:**

_____ _____ _____

_____ _____ _____

_____ _____ _____

_____ _____ _____

_____ _____ _____

_____ _____ _____

PREGNANCIES AND BIRTHS (if applicable)

Approximate Date of Pregnancy:	Date of Birth or End of Pregnancy:	Notes:
_____	_____	_____
		_____
_____	_____	_____
		_____
_____	_____	_____
		_____
_____	_____	_____
		_____

FAMILY ILLNESSES

Relative:	Illness/Cause of Death:	Age:
_____	_____	_____
_____	_____	_____
_____	_____	_____
_____	_____	_____
_____	_____	_____
_____	_____	_____

References

Balch, James F., MD, and Phyllis A. Balch, CNC. *Prescription for Nutritional Healing*, 2nd ed. Garden City Park, NY: Avery Publishing Group, 1997.

Berkow, Robert, MD, ed. in chief. *The Merck Manual of Medical Information*, Home Ed. Whitehouse Station, NJ: Merck & Co., Inc., 1997.

Garrison, Robert, Rph, and Elizabeth Somer. *The Nutrition Desk Reference*, 3rd ed. New Canaan, CT: Keats Publishing, 1997.

Griffith, H, Winter, MD. *Complete Guide to Prescription & Nonprescription Drugs*, 1997 ed. New York, NY: Berkley Publishing Group, 1996.

Gursche, Siegfried, MH. *Encyclopedia of Natural Healing*. Zolton Rona, medical ed. Burnaby, BC: Alive Publishing, Inc., 1997.

Hathcock, John N., PhD. "Vitamin Mineral Safety," for Council for Responsible Nutrition, 1997.

Lieberman, Shari, PhD, and Nancy Bruning. *The Real Vitamin & Mineral Book*, 2nd ed. Garden City Park, NY: Avery Publishing Group, 1997.

Lobay, Douglas, ND. *21st Century Natural Medicine*. Kelowna, BC: Apple Communications, 1992.

Silverman, Harold M., PharmD. *The Pill Book Guide to Safe Drug Use*. New York, NY: Bantam Books, 1989.

Sizer, Frances, and Eleanor Whitney. *Nutrition: Concepts and Controversies*. New York, NY: West Publishing Company, 1994.

References for *Fifty Common Herbs and their Potential Interactions With Regular Drugs* on pages 24 to 41.

[1] American Herbal Pharmacopoeia and Therapeutic Compendium. St. John's Wort Hypericum perforatum. Herbalgram 1997: 40:36. [2] Barnes J. Growing body of data for hypericum extract in depression. InPharma 1996; No. 1058:3-4, Oct 12. [3] Barnett RA. Ginkgo, Ginger, Garlic, Ginseng. Remedy 1996; 33–36, 38–39, Sep/Oct. [4] Becker BN, Greene J, Evanson J, Chidsey G, Stone WU, et. Al. Ginseng-induced diuretic resistance. JAMA 1996; 276: 606–607, Aug 28. [5] Bisset NG (ed). Herbal Drugs and Phytopharmaceuticals. Boca Raton, LA: CRC Press, 1994. [6] Covington TR (ed). The Handbook of Non-Prescription Drugs. Washington, DC: APhA, 1996. [7] Foster S. Ginkgo:Ginkgo biloba, Botanical Series 304. Austin, TX: American Botanical Council: 1991: 1–7. [8] Kassler WJ, Blanc P, Greenblatt R. The use of medicinal herbs by human immunodeficiency virus-infected patients. Arch Intern Med 1991; 151:2281–2288, Nov. [9] Kay MA. Healing with Plants in the American and Mexican West. Tucson, AZ: University of Arizona Press, 1996. [10] Linde K, Ramirez G, Mulrow CD, Pauls A, Weidenhammer W, Melchart D. St. John's wort for depression: an overview

and meta-analysis of randomized clinical trials. BMJ 1996; 313: 253–8, Aug 3. [11] McCann B. Botanical could improve sex life of patients on SSRIs. Drug Topics July 7 1997;33. [12] Osborne F, Chandler F. Sarsaparilla. Canadian Pharmaceutical Journal, 1996. [13] Rawls R. Europe's strong herbal brew. C&EN. 1996: 53–60, Sep 23. [14] Remington KA. A Pharmacist's guide to useful herbal remedies. Calif Pharm 1997; (suppl):1–10 April [15] Review of Natural Products. St.Louis, MO: Facts and Comparisons, 1996. [16] Robbers JE. Speedie MK, Tyler VE. Pharmacognosy and Pharmacobiotechnology. Baltimore, MD: Williams &Wilkins. 1996. [17] Rosenblatt M, Mindel J. Spontaneous hyphema associated with ingestion of Ginkgo biloba extract. (letter). N Engl J Med 1997; 336(15):1108 April 10. [18] Rowin J, Lewis SL. Spontaneous bilateral subdural hematomas associated with chronic Ginkgo biloba ingestion. Neurology 1996; 46: 1775–6. [19] Seligmann J, Cowley G. Sex, Lies, and Garlic. Newsweek 1995; 65–68, Nov. [20] Siciliano AA. Cranberry. HerbalGram 1996; No. 38: 51–54. [21] Singh YN, Blumenthal M. Kava, an overview. HerbalGram 1997; No. 39:33-56. [22] Tyler VE. Herbs of Choice: The therapeutic use of phytomedicinals. New York: Haworth Press, 1994. [23] Tyler VE. What Pharmacists should know about herbal remedies. J APhA 1996; NS36 (1):29–37, Jan. [24] Vogel VJ. American Indian Medicine. Norman, OK: University of Oklahoma Press, 1970. [25] Weiner MA. Earth Medicine, Earth Food. New York: Fawcett Columbine, 1991. [26] Newall CA et al. Herbal Medicines: A Guide for Health Care Professionals. London: The Pharmaceutical Press, 1966. [27] McDaniel HR, et al. An increase in circulating monocyte/macrophages is induced by oral acemannan in HIV-1 patients. Am J Clin Pathol 94: 516–17, 1990.

About the Authors

Robert H. Garrison, Jr., received his pharmacy degree from the University of Washington and his master of arts in education from San Diego State University. He is a health communications specialist whose varied talents range from serving as an executive to publishing a total of fourteen books on nutrition. Among his many accomplishments, he has published *The Essential Guide to Vitamins and Minerals* and co-authored *The Nutrition Desk Reference.* And for twelve years, Garrison served as Editor-in-Chief of *The Nutrition Report,* a leading monthly newsletter covering research in vitamins and minerals.

Garrison has been involved in many aspects of the production of health products for decades. In the late 1970s, he founded Health Media of America, Inc., and served as its President until the early 1990s. This company was the leading provider of new product concepts, marketing, and communication strategies for the major broad line vitamin companies. During that time period, he also co-founded and served as President of the first company to bring the pharmaceutical form of medicinal herbs to United States drug stores.

In 1997, Garrison co-founded Next Pharmaceuticals, Inc., and presently serves as Chairman of the

Board. Next Pharmaceuticals, Inc., is a leading source of new botanical products for expanding self-care choices. Garrison continues to be a leader in health communications. He aims to provide the consumer with up-to-date, well-defined information so that he or she can make responsible, effective decisions that take into consideration the latest in available health products and advice.

Michael Mannion earned his bachelor's degree at Fordham University. He has been a professional medical writer since 1975, working extensively with both conventional and alternative/complementary healthcare issues. Mannion has long been at the cutting edge of health reporting. For example, he wrote on genetic engineering in 1977; hospice care in 1978; and vitamins and cancer in 1980.

From 1977 to 1981, Mannion served as Director of Professional Education Publications and Managing Editor of the American Cancer Society's *Ca-A Cancer Journal for Clinicians*. Throughout the 1980s, he researched and wrote for pharmaceutical-related publications designed for physicians, covering such critical topics as cancer, heart disease, arthritis, stress, depression, anxiety, and women's health. Among his many roles in the field of health literature, Mannion has worked as a writer and editor for PW Communications and other medical publishers, and has written for the New York City Department of Health.

In the 1990s, Mannion turned his interests toward alternative/complementary care. He has worked on projects with the Foundation for Innovation in Medicine; the Institute for Health and Healing; the New York Open Center; Friends of the Institute for Noetic Sciences (board member); Age Wave, Inc.; and the Wilhelm Reich Museum. In addition to *The Pharmacist's Guide to Over-the-Counter and Natural Remedies,* he has authored several works, including *The New American Medicine; How to Help Your Teenager Stop Smoking; 365 Everyday Health Tips—A Daily Guide to Improving Health and Increasing Energy;* and *Project Mindshift.*

Index